FREE Study Skills Videos/DVD Offer

Dear Customer,

Thank you for your purchase from Mometrix! We consider it an honor and a privilege that you have purchased our product and we want to ensure your satisfaction.

As part of our ongoing effort to meet the needs of test takers, we have developed a set of Study Skills Videos that we would like to give you for <u>FREE</u>. These videos cover our *best practices* for getting ready for your exam, from how to use our study materials to how to best prepare for the day of the test.

All that we ask is that you email us with feedback that would describe your experience so far with our product. Good, bad, or indifferent, we want to know what you think!

To get your FREE Study Skills Videos, you can use the **QR code** below, or send us an **email** at studyvideos@mometrix.com with *FREE VIDEOS* in the subject line and the following information in the body of the email:

- The name of the product you purchased.
- Your product rating on a scale of 1-5, with 5 being the highest rating.
- Your feedback. It can be long, short, or anything in between. We just want to know your impressions and experience so far with our product. (Good feedback might include how our study material met your needs and ways we might be able to make it even better. You could highlight features that you found helpful or features that you think we should add.)

If you have any questions or concerns, please don't hesitate to contact me directly.

Thanks again!

Sincerely,

Jay Willis
Vice President
jay.willis@mometrix.com
1-800-673-8175

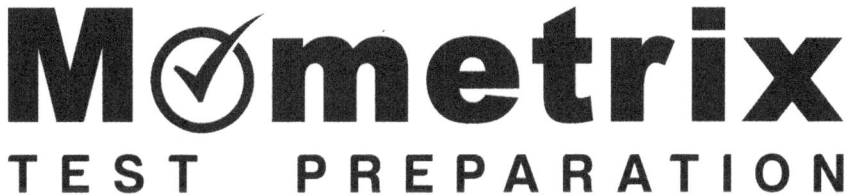

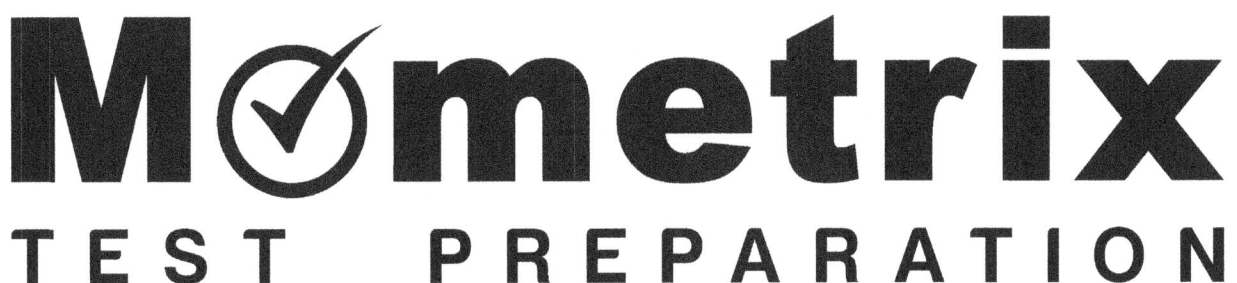

RHIA
Exam Prep Secrets
Study Guide

AHIMA Registered Health Information
Administrator Preparation Review Book

2 Full-Length Practice Tests

Detailed Answer
Explanations

2nd Edition

Copyright © 2023 by Mometrix Media LLC

All rights reserved. This product, or parts thereof, may not be reproduced, stored in a retrieval system, or transmitted in any form or by any means—electronic, mechanical, photocopy, recording, scanning, or other—except for brief quotations in critical reviews or articles, without the prior written permission of the publisher.

Written and edited by the Mometrix Health Information Management Certification Test Team

Printed in the United States of America

This paper meets the requirements of ANSI/NISO Z39.48-1992 (Permanence of Paper).

Mometrix offers volume discount pricing to institutions. For more information or a price quote, please contact our sales department at sales@mometrix.com or 888-248-1219.

Mometrix Media LLC is not affiliated with or endorsed by any official testing organization. All organizational and test names are trademarks of their respective owners.

Paperback
ISBN 13: 978-1-5167-1853-5
ISBN 10: 1-5167-1853-4

Ebook
ISBN 13: 978-1-5167-1917-4
ISBN 10: 1-5167-1917-4

Hardback
ISBN 13: 978-1-5167-1895-5
ISBN 10: 1-5167-1895-X

Dear Future Exam Success Story

First of all, **THANK YOU** for purchasing Mometrix study materials!

Second, congratulations! You are one of the few determined test-takers who are committed to doing whatever it takes to excel on your exam. **You have come to the right place.** We developed these study materials with one goal in mind: to deliver you the information you need in a format that's concise and easy to use.

In addition to optimizing your guide for the content of the test, we've outlined our recommended steps for breaking down the preparation process into small, attainable goals so you can make sure you stay on track.

We've also analyzed the entire test-taking process, identifying the most common pitfalls and showing how you can overcome them and be ready for any curveball the test throws you.

Standardized testing is one of the biggest obstacles on your road to success, which only increases the importance of doing well in the high-pressure, high-stakes environment of test day. Your results on this test could have a significant impact on your future, and this guide provides the information and practical advice to help you achieve your full potential on test day.

Your success is our success

We would love to hear from you! If you would like to share the story of your exam success or if you have any questions or comments in regard to our products, please contact us at **800-673-8175** or **support@mometrix.com**.

Thanks again for your business and we wish you continued success!

Sincerely,
The Mometrix Test Preparation Team

Need more help? Check out our flashcards at:
http://mometrixflashcards.com/RHIA

TABLE OF CONTENTS

INTRODUCTION _____ 1
SECRET KEY #1 – PLAN BIG, STUDY SMALL _____ 2
SECRET KEY #2 – MAKE YOUR STUDYING COUNT _____ 3
SECRET KEY #3 – PRACTICE THE RIGHT WAY _____ 4
SECRET KEY #4 – PACE YOURSELF _____ 6
SECRET KEY #5 – HAVE A PLAN FOR GUESSING _____ 7
TEST-TAKING STRATEGIES _____ 10
INFORMATION GOVERNANCE _____ 15
COMPLIANCE WITH USES AND DISCLOSURES OF PHI _____ 26
DATA ANALYTICS AND INFORMATICS _____ 41
REVENUE MANAGEMENT _____ 57
MANAGEMENT AND LEADERSHIP _____ 66
RHIA PRACTICE TEST #1 _____ 74
ANSWER KEY AND EXPLANATIONS FOR TEST #1 _____ 110
RHIA PRACTICE TEST #2 _____ 125
ANSWER KEY AND EXPLANATIONS FOR TEST #2 _____ 162
HOW TO OVERCOME TEST ANXIETY _____ 186
   CAUSES OF TEST ANXIETY _____ 186
   ELEMENTS OF TEST ANXIETY _____ 187
   EFFECTS OF TEST ANXIETY _____ 187
   PHYSICAL STEPS FOR BEATING TEST ANXIETY _____ 188
   MENTAL STEPS FOR BEATING TEST ANXIETY _____ 189
   STUDY STRATEGY _____ 190
   TEST TIPS _____ 192
   IMPORTANT QUALIFICATION _____ 193
TELL US YOUR STORY _____ 194
ADDITIONAL BONUS MATERIAL _____ 195

Introduction

Thank you for purchasing this resource! You have made the choice to prepare yourself for a test that could have a huge impact on your future, and this guide is designed to help you be fully ready for test day. Obviously, it's important to have a solid understanding of the test material, but you also need to be prepared for the unique environment and stressors of the test, so that you can perform to the best of your abilities.

For this purpose, the first section that appears in this guide is the **Secret Keys**. We've devoted countless hours to meticulously researching what works and what doesn't, and we've boiled down our findings to the five most impactful steps you can take to improve your performance on the test. We start at the beginning with study planning and move through the preparation process, all the way to the testing strategies that will help you get the most out of what you know when you're finally sitting in front of the test.

We recommend that you start preparing for your test as far in advance as possible. However, if you've bought this guide as a last-minute study resource and only have a few days before your test, we recommend that you skip over the first two Secret Keys since they address a long-term study plan.

If you struggle with **test anxiety**, we strongly encourage you to check out our recommendations for how you can overcome it. Test anxiety is a formidable foe, but it can be beaten, and we want to make sure you have the tools you need to defeat it.

Secret Key #1 – Plan Big, Study Small

There's a lot riding on your performance. If you want to ace this test, you're going to need to keep your skills sharp and the material fresh in your mind. You need a plan that lets you review everything you need to know while still fitting in your schedule. We'll break this strategy down into three categories.

Information Organization

Start with the information you already have: the official test outline. From this, you can make a complete list of all the concepts you need to cover before the test. Organize these concepts into groups that can be studied together, and create a list of any related vocabulary you need to learn so you can brush up on any difficult terms. You'll want to keep this vocabulary list handy once you actually start studying since you may need to add to it along the way.

Time Management

Once you have your set of study concepts, decide how to spread them out over the time you have left before the test. Break your study plan into small, clear goals so you have a manageable task for each day and know exactly what you're doing. Then just focus on one small step at a time. When you manage your time this way, you don't need to spend hours at a time studying. Studying a small block of content for a short period each day helps you retain information better and avoid stressing over how much you have left to do. You can relax knowing that you have a plan to cover everything in time. In order for this strategy to be effective though, you have to start studying early and stick to your schedule. Avoid the exhaustion and futility that comes from last-minute cramming!

Study Environment

The environment you study in has a big impact on your learning. Studying in a coffee shop, while probably more enjoyable, is not likely to be as fruitful as studying in a quiet room. It's important to keep distractions to a minimum. You're only planning to study for a short block of time, so make the most of it. Don't pause to check your phone or get up to find a snack. It's also important to **avoid multitasking**. Research has consistently shown that multitasking will make your studying dramatically less effective. Your study area should also be comfortable and well-lit so you don't have the distraction of straining your eyes or sitting on an uncomfortable chair.

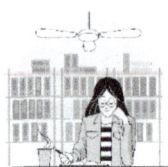

The time of day you study is also important. You want to be rested and alert. Don't wait until just before bedtime. Study when you'll be most likely to comprehend and remember. Even better, if you know what time of day your test will be, set that time aside for study. That way your brain will be used to working on that subject at that specific time and you'll have a better chance of recalling information.

Finally, it can be helpful to team up with others who are studying for the same test. Your actual studying should be done in as isolated an environment as possible, but the work of organizing the information and setting up the study plan can be divided up. In between study sessions, you can discuss with your teammates the concepts that you're all studying and quiz each other on the details. Just be sure that your teammates are as serious about the test as you are. If you find that your study time is being replaced with social time, you might need to find a new team.

Secret Key #2 – Make Your Studying Count

You're devoting a lot of time and effort to preparing for this test, so you want to be absolutely certain it will pay off. This means doing more than just reading the content and hoping you can remember it on test day. It's important to make every minute of study count. There are two main areas you can focus on to make your studying count.

Retention

It doesn't matter how much time you study if you can't remember the material. You need to make sure you are retaining the concepts. To check your retention of the information you're learning, try recalling it at later times with minimal prompting. Try carrying around flashcards and glance at one or two from time to time or ask a friend who's also studying for the test to quiz you.

To enhance your retention, look for ways to put the information into practice so that you can apply it rather than simply recalling it. If you're using the information in practical ways, it will be much easier to remember. Similarly, it helps to solidify a concept in your mind if you're not only reading it to yourself but also explaining it to someone else. Ask a friend to let you teach them about a concept you're a little shaky on (or speak aloud to an imaginary audience if necessary). As you try to summarize, define, give examples, and answer your friend's questions, you'll understand the concepts better and they will stay with you longer. Finally, step back for a big picture view and ask yourself how each piece of information fits with the whole subject. When you link the different concepts together and see them working together as a whole, it's easier to remember the individual components.

Finally, practice showing your work on any multi-step problems, even if you're just studying. Writing out each step you take to solve a problem will help solidify the process in your mind, and you'll be more likely to remember it during the test.

Modality

Modality simply refers to the means or method by which you study. Choosing a study modality that fits your own individual learning style is crucial. No two people learn best in exactly the same way, so it's important to know your strengths and use them to your advantage.

For example, if you learn best by visualization, focus on visualizing a concept in your mind and draw an image or a diagram. Try color-coding your notes, illustrating them, or creating symbols that will trigger your mind to recall a learned concept. If you learn best by hearing or discussing information, find a study partner who learns the same way or read aloud to yourself. Think about how to put the information in your own words. Imagine that you are giving a lecture on the topic and record yourself so you can listen to it later.

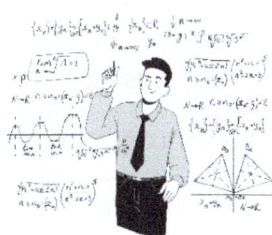

For any learning style, flashcards can be helpful. Organize the information so you can take advantage of spare moments to review. Underline key words or phrases. Use different colors for different categories. Mnemonic devices (such as creating a short list in which every item starts with the same letter) can also help with retention. Find what works best for you and use it to store the information in your mind most effectively and easily.

Secret Key #3 – Practice the Right Way

Your success on test day depends not only on how many hours you put into preparing, but also on whether you prepared the right way. It's good to check along the way to see if your studying is paying off. One of the most effective ways to do this is by taking practice tests to evaluate your progress. Practice tests are useful because they show exactly where you need to improve. Every time you take a practice test, pay special attention to these three groups of questions:

- The questions you got wrong
- The questions you had to guess on, even if you guessed right
- The questions you found difficult or slow to work through

This will show you exactly what your weak areas are, and where you need to devote more study time. Ask yourself why each of these questions gave you trouble. Was it because you didn't understand the material? Was it because you didn't remember the vocabulary? Do you need more repetitions on this type of question to build speed and confidence? Dig into those questions and figure out how you can strengthen your weak areas as you go back to review the material.

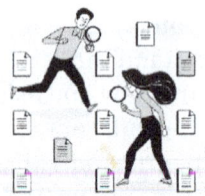

Additionally, many practice tests have a section explaining the answer choices. It can be tempting to read the explanation and think that you now have a good understanding of the concept. However, an explanation likely only covers part of the question's broader context. Even if the explanation makes perfect sense, **go back and investigate** every concept related to the question until you're positive you have a thorough understanding.

As you go along, keep in mind that the practice test is just that: practice. Memorizing these questions and answers will not be very helpful on the actual test because it is unlikely to have any of the same exact questions. If you only know the right answers to the sample questions, you won't be prepared for the real thing. **Study the concepts** until you understand them fully, and then you'll be able to answer any question that shows up on the test.

It's important to wait on the practice tests until you're ready. If you take a test on your first day of study, you may be overwhelmed by the amount of material covered and how much you need to learn. Work up to it gradually.

On test day, you'll need to be prepared for answering questions, managing your time, and using the test-taking strategies you've learned. It's a lot to balance, like a mental marathon that will have a big impact on your future. Like training for a marathon, you'll need to start slowly and work your way up. When test day arrives, you'll be ready.

Start with the strategies you've read in the first two Secret Keys—plan your course and study in the way that works best for you. If you have time, consider using multiple study resources to get different approaches to the same concepts. It can be helpful to see difficult concepts from more than one angle. Then find a good source for practice tests. Many times, the test website will suggest potential study resources or provide sample tests.

Practice Test Strategy

If you're able to find at least three practice tests, we recommend this strategy:

UNTIMED AND OPEN-BOOK PRACTICE

Take the first test with no time constraints and with your notes and study guide handy. Take your time and focus on applying the strategies you've learned.

TIMED AND OPEN-BOOK PRACTICE

Take the second practice test open-book as well, but set a timer and practice pacing yourself to finish in time.

TIMED AND CLOSED-BOOK PRACTICE

Take any other practice tests as if it were test day. Set a timer and put away your study materials. Sit at a table or desk in a quiet room, imagine yourself at the testing center, and answer questions as quickly and accurately as possible.

Keep repeating timed and closed-book tests on a regular basis until you run out of practice tests or it's time for the actual test. Your mind will be ready for the schedule and stress of test day, and you'll be able to focus on recalling the material you've learned.

Secret Key #4 – Pace Yourself

Once you're fully prepared for the material on the test, your biggest challenge on test day will be managing your time. Just knowing that the clock is ticking can make you panic even if you have plenty of time left. Work on pacing yourself so you can build confidence against the time constraints of the exam. Pacing is a difficult skill to master, especially in a high-pressure environment, so **practice is vital**.

Set time expectations for your pace based on how much time is available. For example, if a section has 60 questions and the time limit is 30 minutes, you know you have to average 30 seconds or less per question in order to answer them all. Although 30 seconds is the hard limit, set 25 seconds per question as your goal, so you reserve extra time to spend on harder questions. When you budget extra time for the harder questions, you no longer have any reason to stress when those questions take longer to answer.

Don't let this time expectation distract you from working through the test at a calm, steady pace, but keep it in mind so you don't spend too much time on any one question. Recognize that taking extra time on one question you don't understand may keep you from answering two that you do understand later in the test. If your time limit for a question is up and you're still not sure of the answer, mark it and move on, and come back to it later if the time and the test format allow. If the testing format doesn't allow you to return to earlier questions, just make an educated guess; then put it out of your mind and move on.

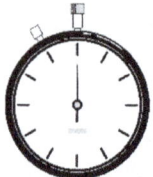

On the easier questions, be careful not to rush. It may seem wise to hurry through them so you have more time for the challenging ones, but it's not worth missing one if you know the concept and just didn't take the time to read the question fully. Work efficiently but make sure you understand the question and have looked at all of the answer choices, since more than one may seem right at first.

Even if you're paying attention to the time, you may find yourself a little behind at some point. You should speed up to get back on track, but do so wisely. Don't panic; just take a few seconds less on each question until you're caught up. Don't guess without thinking, but do look through the answer choices and eliminate any you know are wrong. If you can get down to two choices, it is often worthwhile to guess from those. Once you've chosen an answer, move on and don't dwell on any that you skipped or had to hurry through. If a question was taking too long, chances are it was one of the harder ones, so you weren't as likely to get it right anyway.

On the other hand, if you find yourself getting ahead of schedule, it may be beneficial to slow down a little. The more quickly you work, the more likely you are to make a careless mistake that will affect your score. You've budgeted time for each question, so don't be afraid to spend that time. Practice an efficient but careful pace to get the most out of the time you have.

Secret Key #5 – Have a Plan for Guessing

When you're taking the test, you may find yourself stuck on a question. Some of the answer choices seem better than others, but you don't see the one answer choice that is obviously correct. What do you do?

The scenario described above is very common, yet most test takers have not effectively prepared for it. Developing and practicing a plan for guessing may be one of the single most effective uses of your time as you get ready for the exam.

In developing your plan for guessing, there are three questions to address:

- When should you start the guessing process?
- How should you narrow down the choices?
- Which answer should you choose?

When to Start the Guessing Process

Unless your plan for guessing is to select C every time (which, despite its merits, is not what we recommend), you need to leave yourself enough time to apply your answer elimination strategies. Since you have a limited amount of time for each question, that means that if you're going to give yourself the best shot at guessing correctly, you have to decide quickly whether or not you will guess.

Of course, the best-case scenario is that you don't have to guess at all, so first, see if you can answer the question based on your knowledge of the subject and basic reasoning skills. Focus on the key words in the question and try to jog your memory of related topics. Give yourself a chance to bring the knowledge to mind, but once you realize that you don't have (or you can't access) the knowledge you need to answer the question, it's time to start the guessing process.

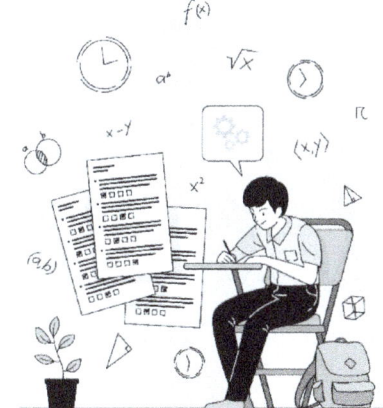

It's almost always better to start the guessing process too early than too late. It only takes a few seconds to remember something and answer the question from knowledge. Carefully eliminating wrong answer choices takes longer. Plus, going through the process of eliminating answer choices can actually help jog your memory.

Summary: Start the guessing process as soon as you decide that you can't answer the question based on your knowledge.

How to Narrow Down the Choices

The next chapter in this book (**Test-Taking Strategies**) includes a wide range of strategies for how to approach questions and how to look for answer choices to eliminate. You will definitely want to read those carefully, practice them, and figure out which ones work best for you. Here though, we're going to address a mindset rather than a particular strategy.

Your odds of guessing an answer correctly depend on how many options you are choosing from.

Number of options left	5	4	3	2	1
Odds of guessing correctly	20%	25%	33%	50%	100%

You can see from this chart just how valuable it is to be able to eliminate incorrect answers and make an educated guess, but there are two things that many test takers do that cause them to miss out on the benefits of guessing:

- Accidentally eliminating the correct answer
- Selecting an answer based on an impression

We'll look at the first one here, and the second one in the next section.

To avoid accidentally eliminating the correct answer, we recommend a thought exercise called **the $5 challenge**. In this challenge, you only eliminate an answer choice from contention if you are willing to bet $5 on it being wrong. Why $5? Five dollars is a small but not insignificant amount of money. It's an amount you could afford to lose but wouldn't want to throw away. And while losing

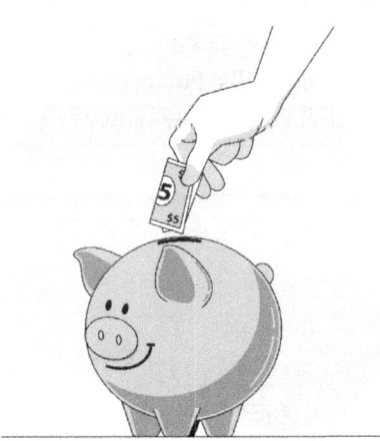

$5 once might not hurt too much, doing it twenty times will set you back $100. In the same way, each small decision you make—eliminating a choice here, guessing on a question there—won't by itself impact your score very much, but when you put them all together, they can make a big difference. By holding each answer choice elimination decision to a higher standard, you can reduce the risk of accidentally eliminating the correct answer.

The $5 challenge can also be applied in a positive sense: If you are willing to bet $5 that an answer choice *is* correct, go ahead and mark it as correct.

Summary: Only eliminate an answer choice if you are willing to bet $5 that it is wrong.

Which Answer to Choose

You're taking the test. You've run into a hard question and decided you'll have to guess. You've eliminated all the answer choices you're willing to bet $5 on. Now you have to pick an answer. Why do we even need to talk about this? Why can't you just pick whichever one you feel like when the time comes?

The answer to these questions is that if you don't come into the test with a plan, you'll rely on your impression to select an answer choice, and if you do that, you risk falling into a trap. The test writers know that everyone who takes their test will be guessing on some of the questions, so they intentionally write wrong answer choices to seem plausible. You still have to pick an answer though, and if the wrong answer choices are designed to look right, how can you ever be sure that you're not falling for their trap? The best solution we've found to this dilemma is to take the decision out of your hands entirely. Here is the process we recommend:

Once you've eliminated any choices that you are confident (willing to bet $5) are wrong, select the first remaining choice as your answer.

Whether you choose to select the first remaining choice, the second, or the last, the important thing is that you use some preselected standard. Using this approach guarantees that you will not be enticed into selecting an answer choice that looks right, because you are not basing your decision on how the answer choices look.

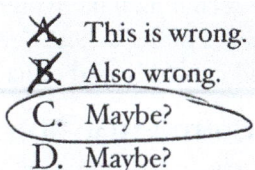

This is not meant to make you question your knowledge. Instead, it is to help you recognize the difference between your knowledge and your impressions. There's a huge difference between thinking an answer is right because of what you know, and thinking an answer is right because it looks or sounds like it should be right.

Summary: To ensure that your selection is appropriately random, make a predetermined selection from among all answer choices you have not eliminated.

Test-Taking Strategies

This section contains a list of test-taking strategies that you may find helpful as you work through the test. By taking what you know and applying logical thought, you can maximize your chances of answering any question correctly!

It is very important to realize that every question is different and every person is different: no single strategy will work on every question, and no single strategy will work for every person. That's why we've included all of them here, so you can try them out and determine which ones work best for different types of questions and which ones work best for you.

Question Strategies

☑ READ CAREFULLY

Read the question and the answer choices carefully. Don't miss the question because you misread the terms. You have plenty of time to read each question thoroughly and make sure you understand what is being asked. Yet a happy medium must be attained, so don't waste too much time. You must read carefully and efficiently.

☑ CONTEXTUAL CLUES

Look for contextual clues. If the question includes a word you are not familiar with, look at the immediate context for some indication of what the word might mean. Contextual clues can often give you all the information you need to decipher the meaning of an unfamiliar word. Even if you can't determine the meaning, you may be able to narrow down the possibilities enough to make a solid guess at the answer to the question.

☑ PREFIXES

If you're having trouble with a word in the question or answer choices, try dissecting it. Take advantage of every clue that the word might include. Prefixes can be a huge help. Usually, they allow you to determine a basic meaning. *Pre-* means before, *post-* means after, *pro-* is positive, *de-* is negative. From prefixes, you can get an idea of the general meaning of the word and try to put it into context.

☑ HEDGE WORDS

Watch out for critical hedge words, such as *likely, may, can, sometimes, often, almost, mostly, usually, generally, rarely,* and *sometimes*. Question writers insert these hedge phrases to cover every possibility. Often an answer choice will be wrong simply because it leaves no room for exception. Be on guard for answer choices that have definitive words such as *exactly* and *always*.

☑ SWITCHBACK WORDS

Stay alert for *switchbacks*. These are the words and phrases frequently used to alert you to shifts in thought. The most common switchback words are *but, although,* and *however*. Others include *nevertheless, on the other hand, even though, while, in spite of, despite,* and *regardless of*. Switchback words are important to catch because they can change the direction of the question or an answer choice.

10

⊘ FACE VALUE

When in doubt, use common sense. Accept the situation in the problem at face value. Don't read too much into it. These problems will not require you to make wild assumptions. If you have to go beyond creativity and warp time or space in order to have an answer choice fit the question, then you should move on and consider the other answer choices. These are normal problems rooted in reality. The applicable relationship or explanation may not be readily apparent, but it is there for you to figure out. Use your common sense to interpret anything that isn't clear.

Answer Choice Strategies

⊘ ANSWER SELECTION

The most thorough way to pick an answer choice is to identify and eliminate wrong answers until only one is left, then confirm it is the correct answer. Sometimes an answer choice may immediately seem right, but be careful. The test writers will usually put more than one reasonable answer choice on each question, so take a second to read all of them and make sure that the other choices are not equally obvious. As long as you have time left, it is better to read every answer choice than to pick the first one that looks right without checking the others.

⊘ ANSWER CHOICE FAMILIES

An answer choice family consists of two (in rare cases, three) answer choices that are very similar in construction and cannot all be true at the same time. If you see two answer choices that are direct opposites or parallels, one of them is usually the correct answer. For instance, if one answer choice says that quantity x increases and another either says that quantity x decreases (opposite) or says that quantity y increases (parallel), then those answer choices would fall into the same family. An answer choice that doesn't match the construction of the answer choice family is more likely to be incorrect. Most questions will not have answer choice families, but when they do appear, you should be prepared to recognize them.

⊘ ELIMINATE ANSWERS

Eliminate answer choices as soon as you realize they are wrong, but make sure you consider all possibilities. If you are eliminating answer choices and realize that the last one you are left with is also wrong, don't panic. Start over and consider each choice again. There may be something you missed the first time that you will realize on the second pass.

⊘ AVOID FACT TRAPS

Don't be distracted by an answer choice that is factually true but doesn't answer the question. You are looking for the choice that answers the question. Stay focused on what the question is asking for so you don't accidentally pick an answer that is true but incorrect. Always go back to the question and make sure the answer choice you've selected actually answers the question and is not merely a true statement.

⊘ EXTREME STATEMENTS

In general, you should avoid answers that put forth extreme actions as standard practice or proclaim controversial ideas as established fact. An answer choice that states the "process should be used in certain situations, if…" is much more likely to be correct than one that states the "process should be discontinued completely." The first is a calm rational statement and doesn't even make a definitive, uncompromising stance, using a hedge word *if* to provide wiggle room, whereas the second choice is far more extreme.

⊘ Benchmark

As you read through the answer choices and you come across one that seems to answer the question well, mentally select that answer choice. This is not your final answer, but it's the one that will help you evaluate the other answer choices. The one that you selected is your benchmark or standard for judging each of the other answer choices. Every other answer choice must be compared to your benchmark. That choice is correct until proven otherwise by another answer choice beating it. If you find a better answer, then that one becomes your new benchmark. Once you've decided that no other choice answers the question as well as your benchmark, you have your final answer.

⊘ Predict the Answer

Before you even start looking at the answer choices, it is often best to try to predict the answer. When you come up with the answer on your own, it is easier to avoid distractions and traps because you will know exactly what to look for. The right answer choice is unlikely to be word-for-word what you came up with, but it should be a close match. Even if you are confident that you have the right answer, you should still take the time to read each option before moving on.

General Strategies

⊘ Tough Questions

If you are stumped on a problem or it appears too hard or too difficult, don't waste time. Move on! Remember though, if you can quickly check for obviously incorrect answer choices, your chances of guessing correctly are greatly improved. Before you completely give up, at least try to knock out a couple of possible answers. Eliminate what you can and then guess at the remaining answer choices before moving on.

⊘ Check Your Work

Since you will probably not know every term listed and the answer to every question, it is important that you get credit for the ones that you do know. Don't miss any questions through careless mistakes. If at all possible, try to take a second to look back over your answer selection and make sure you've selected the correct answer choice and haven't made a costly careless mistake (such as marking an answer choice that you didn't mean to mark). This quick double check should more than pay for itself in caught mistakes for the time it costs.

⊘ Pace Yourself

It's easy to be overwhelmed when you're looking at a page full of questions; your mind is confused and full of random thoughts, and the clock is ticking down faster than you would like. Calm down and maintain the pace that you have set for yourself. Especially as you get down to the last few minutes of the test, don't let the small numbers on the clock make you panic. As long as you are on track by monitoring your pace, you are guaranteed to have time for each question.

⊘ Don't Rush

It is very easy to make errors when you are in a hurry. Maintaining a fast pace in answering questions is pointless if it makes you miss questions that you would have gotten right otherwise. Test writers like to include distracting information and wrong answers that seem right. Taking a little extra time to avoid careless mistakes can make all the difference in your test score. Find a pace that allows you to be confident in the answers that you select.

⊘ Keep Moving

Panicking will not help you pass the test, so do your best to stay calm and keep moving. Taking deep breaths and going through the answer elimination steps you practiced can help to break through a stress barrier and keep your pace.

Final Notes

The combination of a solid foundation of content knowledge and the confidence that comes from practicing your plan for applying that knowledge is the key to maximizing your performance on test day. As your foundation of content knowledge is built up and strengthened, you'll find that the strategies included in this chapter become more and more effective in helping you quickly sift through the distractions and traps of the test to isolate the correct answer.

Now that you're preparing to move forward into the test content chapters of this book, be sure to keep your goal in mind. As you read, think about how you will be able to apply this information on the test. If you've already seen sample questions for the test and you have an idea of the question format and style, try to come up with questions of your own that you can answer based on what you're reading. This will give you valuable practice applying your knowledge in the same ways you can expect to on test day.

Good luck and good studying!

Information Governance

INTEGRITY OF HEALTH DATA

DATA INTEGRITY

Although there is a quantitative piece to data integrity, **data integrity** also entails security measures put in place that ensure that data are not altered, modified, or deleted either accidentally or with malicious intent. Consider the following scenario: a patient experienced an adverse reaction to a medication. The nurse who administered the drug accesses her entry in the medical record and alters the dosage to the correct dosage. This is an extreme example, but it displays the importance of data integrity. Integrity measures may include ensuring that every entry into the medical records is a locked, signed entry or document; that versioning of documents is permitted and accessible; or, for paper records, that entries are written in ink. Inadvertent errors will occur, so ensuring that proper error-correction policies and procedures are in place will help maintain data integrity. Data integrity assists leadership when analyzing best practices, performance improvement (PI) initiatives, or regulation of corrective actions.

DATA CORRECTION OR VERSIONING

An important aspect of data integrity is to ensure that the data visible to the reader are true, accurate, and validated by the author. When an error is identified, a correction is made by editing the document or entry, which will then create a new version of the same document or entry. Consider the following scenario: a staff member makes an edit to her daily nursing assessment. But after completing her edit, she can delete the previous version. Consider the repercussions should a patient event occur; it will be unclear what she edited or omitted from the first version. The previous version should be hidden and archived within the EMR databases. It is important that all versions of documents and entries be accessible in the event of a lawsuit or other discovery process. The most recent locked and signed version will be visible and will be considered the legal record. Ensuring that all document and entry corrections are made legitimately and under the organization's policies and procedures helps to maintain the overall record and data integrity.

DATA INTEGRITY CONSTRAINTS

Data integrity constraints are conditions in which a field in an EMR is programmed and how it will store data. For example, a date field will only contain numeric characters and the field must be in the MM/DD/YYYY date format. Similarly, a last-name field may only contain alphabetic characters with a legal value of 12. A **legal value** is a data integrity condition stating the minimum and maximum entry that a field can house, so a last name of 13 characters would result in an error message. Consider the following scenario: a new EMR program has a medical record number (MRN) field with a legal value set of 00001 to 99999, gambling that it will be many years before the facility reaches an MRN of 99999. Data constraints ensure that the data entered in those fields are consistent, function the same throughout the EMR, and when entered in error would produce the same error messages; it also allows for easy staff training, data abstraction, and reporting.

ARCHIVING OF PROTECTED HEALTH INFORMATION (PHI)

Record archiving is the practice of categorizing, boxing, and storing records for an extended period. Record retention and archival practices are required by law when securing and storing medical records. PHI will be requested from Health Information Management (HIM) departments for various reasons for years to come, and it is critical for organizations to have policies related to archival practices. Consider the following scenario: an HIM clerk requests an 11-year-old medical record from off-site storage. The record is inaccessible because the records were not categorized or indexed appropriately 11 years ago. As a result, unless the HIM clerk can properly identify the box that the record is housed in, it is unlikely they will find it without an extensive search. Maintaining uniformity when logging records for archiving is critical to identify the location of that record later. Additionally, maintaining the data integrity of the logbooks will ensure that the records are maintained in confidential and access-limited conditions.

DATA INTEGRITY AND RELEASE OF INFORMATION (ROI)

Release of information (ROI) is instrumental in the overall business practices of a healthcare organization and HIM department. PHI is released for many different purposes: educational, coordination of care, legal, community support, custody, etc. Not only is data integrity required for record management, it strongly ties into ROI because the medical record is a tool used for many of these high-risk areas. Consider the following scenario: an ancillary healthcare site requests records on Jon Jones. The HIM retrieves and faxes medical records on John Jones. Or consider this: an HIM clerk mails the original progress note rather than a photocopy; as a result, the original notes were compromised and altered. Without data integrity policies and procedures, strict constraints and training could have detrimental effects on patient care, placement of educational or community services, or overall inaccurate decision making based on receiving the incorrect PHI.

REQUIRED CLINICAL DATA ELEMENTS FOR QUALITY REPORTING
LENGTH OF STAY (LOS)

A common HIM and healthcare statistic is the average length of stay (ALOS). The **length of stay (LOS)** for a patient is the difference between the discharge date and the admission date, and it can assist in analyzing costs for hospital stays. For instance, suppose Mary was admitted on February 20, 2020, and discharged February 24, 2020. Her LOS is 4 days. The discharge date is not routinely counted because the patient is discharged prior to midnight; a bed day is calculated at midnight.

Consider the following scenario: senior leaders seek the ALOS for their adult populations whose primary diagnosis is type 1 diabetes.

At a minimum, the admission and discharge dates are needed to calculate the LOS and average them together to find the final ALOS. Additional data elements may be used to identify the ALOS for any patient population, e.g., ALOS by patient age, gender, unit, program, diagnosis, or by physician, etc.

IMPLEMENTING AN AUDIT

An **audit** is a review or analysis of a record to ensure that policies and procedures are being followed. Auditing a new initiative should include completion and quality audits to be sure that the information needed is present, legible, and reliable. Identifying an **audit sample**, or how many records will be reviewed, will depend on the accessibility of the information. In other words, it depends on whether the information can be easily extracted from an electronic medical record (EMR) or if the information must be pulled manually from paper records.

Consider the following scenario: senior management would like monthly statistics on a newly implemented process dealing with pre- and post-procedure pain scores. In this scenario, the audit begins by identifying whether the pre- and post-procedure pain score data are collated from an electronic source or by pulling the data from a paper medication administration record. Either audit will consist of identifying which pain medications or nonpharmacological pain interventions were administered. Then taking the difference between the pre- and post-procedure pain scores will help identify whether a pain intervention was effective or not.

Patient Census Bed Day

A patient census day, also known as a **bed day,** is the number of beds that a hospital has for any given 24-hour period, whether that bed is occupied or vacant. A hospital census is taken at midnight in accordance with the Centers for Medicare & Medicaid Services' requirements for the level of care and reimbursement that hospitals must follow. The **percentage of occupancy** is the percentage of occupied beds against the total number of licensed beds. For example, ABC Hospital is licensed for 88 beds. In the month of September in which there are 30 days, the hospital has 2,640 possible bed census days. ABC Hospital ended the month of September with 2,580 bed days. This would indicate that the hospital has an average bed day each day of September of 86 or 97.7% occupancy. Because the occupancy is not at 100%, it would indicate that it had open beds available during the month of September.

Readmission Rates

Readmission rates are a measure of the number of unique patients who return to the facility. Typically, readmission rates are measured at 7, 14, and 30 days. Readmission rates are analyzed to improve patient flow throughout the organization, monitor utilization of services and supplies, and identify areas of clinical improvements to help reduce patient readmissions, as well as other clinical or administrative indicators. For example, a high 7-day readmission rate would indicate that the same patients keep returning for services; leadership may want to review discharge planning practices. A high 30-day readmission may indicate a situational or environmental precipitant that may or may not be controllable. Measuring readmission rates and maintaining low rates are factors that could be used for budgetary or contractual negotiations with payers.

Patient Outcomes and Satisfaction Data

Patient outcomes are a clinical measurement of the quality of patient care. For example, a patient fills out a symptom rating scale at admission, and the patient is asked to fill out the same rating scale for the same symptoms at discharge. The difference in the scores can be measured to see how well the organization took care of the patient's symptoms. **Satisfaction** scores are additional measurements taken from surveys, scales, or questionnaires that help leadership identify how well the organization and its staff are performing and how pleased the patient is with the treatment, facility, cleanliness, or other quality indicators. Consider the pain graph below, which displays admission and discharge pain scores. The graph would suggest that patients with stomach, head, and chest pain improved over the course of their hospitalization whereas patients with arm pain worsened over their hospitalizations. The second graph is an example of a patient satisfaction result showing that more patients are satisfied with staff professionalism than are dissatisfied.

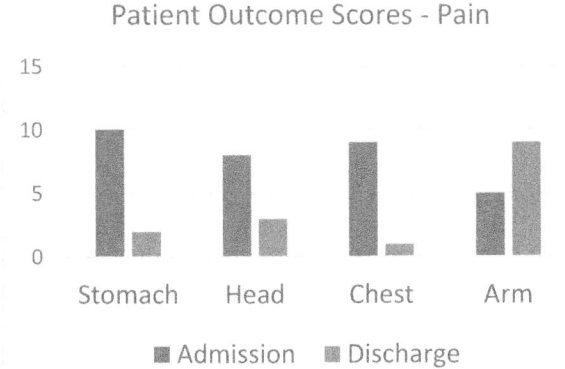
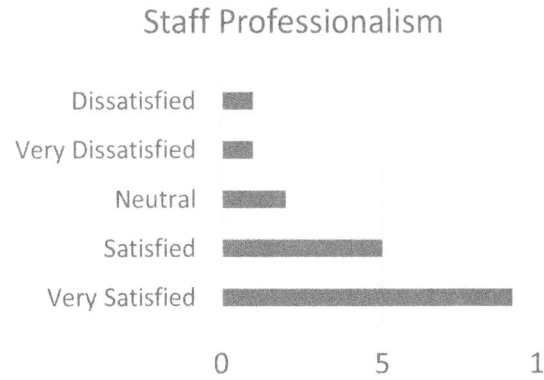

DATA DICTIONARY STANDARDIZATION POLICIES
DATA DICTIONARY

A data dictionary is a list of data elements, definitions, or data types and a description of how the piece of data will be used. Consider the following example as a simplified data dictionary: a typical HIM data dictionary has a master patient index (MPI). In an MPI, there will be a last-name field that is a text-only field made up of a certain number of only alphabetic characters. It will have the data definition of being the patient's birth last name or maiden name if now married or his or her legally changed last name. Data dictionaries can be built into a preexisting EMR database because some fields are predefined by industry or social standards. Other data dictionaries built outside the framework of the system design are completed when the entity wants to control the data nomenclature, data types, and descriptions prior to designing the functionality of each field within the EMR. It can be an extensive project, but maintaining a complete and accurate data dictionary is key to controlling the quality of data in the EMR.

STANDARDIZATION

HIM healthcare standards and best practices have already set the framework for a successful data dictionary, for example, how data interact with other data or fields within a database. Consider the following scenarios: a patient cannot be given an admission date until the admission event is tied to a program or a patient cannot be put into a program until a bed assignment is available. When one or several conditions or events depend on or will be associated with the success of a previous condition or event, it is called **relationship representation**. Relationships are designed, defined, and set up in a data dictionary and are the standardized framework and fundamental build of most data dictionaries. The three different relationships are as follows:

- **One-to-one:** one event is associated to only one event.
- **One-to-many:** one event is associated to many other events.
- **Many-to-many:** many events are associated to many other events.

DATA DICTIONARY DEVELOPMENT

Because a data dictionary is one of the fundamental building blocks of an application used by an organization, it is critical to ensure that the development of a data dictionary is thorough and is in line with organizational policies and practices. Without a well-built data dictionary, the result and output of reports as well as data being pulled from a system (such as an EMR) will be incomplete, inaccurate, and unreliable. The first step to successfully developing a successful data dictionary is to define the scope. In other words, will the data dictionary apply to only one application, one unit of a facility, or the entire facility as a whole? Next, define the interdisciplinary team who will bring the clinical and administrative perspectives to the project development. Lastly, the project team will want to identify priorities and a timeline. Ensuring that these steps are taken means that a comprehensive, inclusive, and universal data dictionary will be used and adapted by all disciplinary programs across the hospital because all had a hand in its development.

DATABASE LIFE CYCLE (DBLC)

According to the American Health Information Management Association (AHIMA), a **database life cycle (DBLC)** is a system consisting of several phases that represent the usual life of a database, i.e., the stages that a database goes through from start to finish. That cycle usually consists of the following steps: initial study, design, implementation, testing and evaluation, operation and maintenance, and evaluation. The rollout and life cycle must be carefully outlined and handled because one stage may be dependent on the success of the previous one. Understanding a DBLC is critical when an organization wishes to implement a new system or manage a full database. A DBLC development team will consist of several people who have expertise in each of the various stages and continue to work the database throughout its full cycle.

Data Mining

Data mining is an automated process in which data are extracted from a source and collected and aggregated into meaningful patterns. Data collected through data mining are routinely classified into one of the following categories: **patient-centric**, meaning the data are centered around patient information; **aggregate**, meaning the data are based on performance or utilization; **transform-based data** are used for management and strategic planning from organizational leadership; and, finally, **comparative data** or data used for research and outcome purposes. Data mining can be beneficial to the HIM field because it helps identify positive or negative documentation trends, behaviors and billing errors, and it outlines the distribution of services. Consider the following scenario: an HIM director uses the data mining technique to pull 100% of the primary diagnosis codes from all patient files for the past 5 years. Those data are then compared to the utilization of services within the organization. Data mining is a critical activity for maintaining and analyzing large amounts of data for strategic decision making.

Data Standards Based on Organizational Policy
Data Standard

Data standards are the best practices or industry approved methods that set the criteria for how data or information is gathered, used, stored, or shared, either inside or outside the organization. Data standards should be set to all medias in which PHI is used or stored. That could be the EMR, medication dispensing or other pharmacy programs, record archival systems, radiology, or other imaging systems. Consider the following scenario: one hospital's radiology film is stored electronically in their ancillary radiology department's program, not in the EMR, whereas another hospital chooses to pull the images out of their radiology program in order to move, store, use, and disclose the images right out of the EMR. Each entity will be required to develop their own data standards around how the radiology films are handled and enforce it through organizational policies and procedures. Data standardization also allows for data consistency and uniformity because entities have many ancillary programs all interfacing with the home EMR.

Nomenclature

Nomenclature is a pre-established set of terms, words, or naming conventions. For example, a medical hospital may choose to call the person seeking treatment a *patient*, whereas a psychiatric hospital may choose to call the patient a *client*. Although there is already an established list of industry and socially acceptable terms, it will be up to the organization of which nomenclature they adopt. Depending on the context, the term used for a medical doctor could be attending physician, psychiatrist, prescriber, surgeon, consultant, specialist, primary care provider, or internist. It is important to follow the organization's structure and policy regarding nomenclature for clarity in communication, continuity of care, political correctness, and even marketing because it is how the facility wants to be represented.

Incident Management Program

Collecting data related to incidents is an important activity to ensure that organizational quality-of-care standards, practices, and expectations are met. Because there are state and federal incident reporting requirements, it is critical to have data standards in place related to what and how incidents are reported through the organization. Routinely, patient, employee, visitor, and medication error incidents are reported and monitored. Consider the following scenario: ABC Hospital measures patient incidents related to adverse drug reactions, employee incidents related to needlesticks, and visitor incidents related to falls. Striving to maintain a staff culture of reporting will increase the success of an incident management program. The following two graphs depict how incident data could be displayed for monitoring activities. Graphing incident data will offer a visual depiction that will identify high-risk areas of an organization, as well as assist with improving the overall quality of care patterns.

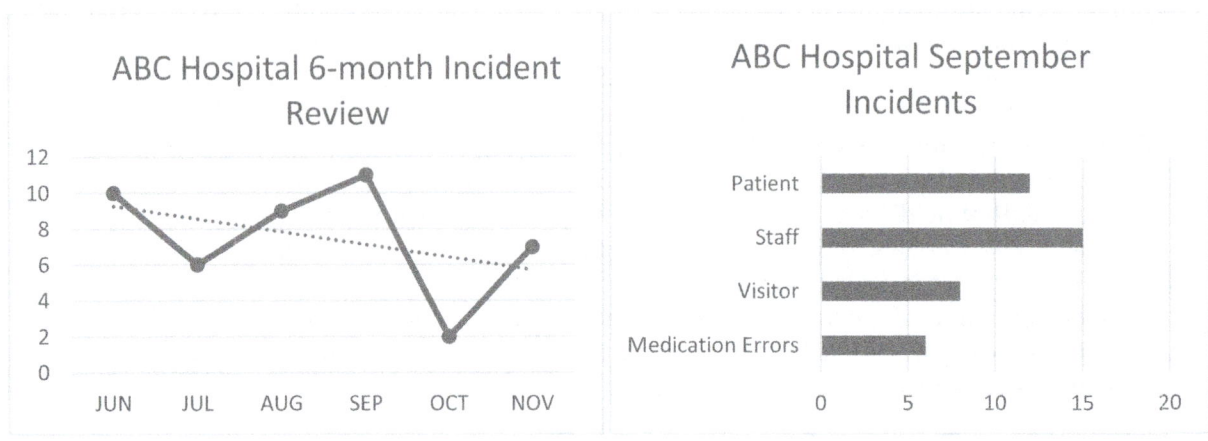

IMPORTANCE OF DATA STANDARDS

Data collected for the purpose of analysis and business decision-making processes should be reliable and accurate. When data are converted to statistical information, it is critical to ensure that the source documentation is held to the organization's policies and procedures. An example of this would be requiring all nursing staff to document vital signs the same way, with the same format, and using the same data fields in the EMR. Encouraging this standardization will ensure that vital signs are not fragmented or illegible throughout the record. The medical record is routinely the source documentation from which all statistical and patient analysis documentation is derived from. Having data standards will ensure that the data pulled for statistical or other analytical reviews are highly accurate and the organization is effective in turning those data into numbers. This in turn helps data to be more readily converted to numerical pictures, in other words, functional data will assist in achieving, monitoring, or creating business or patient care initiatives.

FORM INVENTORY

A form inventory is the collection of titles, purpose, identification, format, and status or versioning information of the forms used by an organization. For example, all pediatric forms are listed with their description and purpose and sorted in the list by a form number. A **form number** is a method of unique identification that is assigned to a form. The following grid could be a sample section of a form inventory.

Form No.	Title	Purpose	Media	Version, Revision Date
ABC-001	PRN Pain Medex	Medication Administration	Paper	v1, 9/12/2001
ABC-002	Vital Sign Flowsheet	Patient Care	EMR	v2, 2/9/1999
ABC-003	Nursing Fall Risk Assessment	Assessment	EMR	v1, 7/25/2020
ABC-004	Observation Order Form	MD Orders	EMR	v1, 7/25/2020

In general, a hospital's form committee approves all forms before they are implemented. Assigning a form number is the final step in the approval process, and once it is done, the form is considered an approved legal medical record form and can be used by staff. If a form number is missing, it would indicate to staff that the form has not been through the proper steps and approval processes. Even if a hospital has a fully electronic medical record, disaster preparedness would require downtime forms. Therefore, the form inventory will assist in organizational record uniformity and data standardizations.

DATA ANALYSIS TO INFORM MANAGEMENT
DATA ANALYSIS

Data analysis is the practice of interpreting data collected by an organization and converting them to meaningful information. Analyzed information can be used to identify PI initiatives, financial needs, staffing, or patient trends as well as assist in the overall strategic planning of the organization. Common data elements to analyze at a healthcare facility include the following:

- length of stay
- number of admissions
- number of discharges
- readmission rates
- no-show rates
- dollar amounts in accounts receivable

Analyzing one or many of these data elements together will help in identifying the successes and weaknesses in an organization. For example, if a provider has higher readmission rates than another provider, that could result in a quality performance initiative or a disciplinary action because it could indicate that the provider has not provided quality care during the initial patient stay. Organizations will collect an enormous amount of clinical and administrative facility statistics as well as financial data to monitor their overall success and functioning.

DATA ANALYSIS AND BUDGETING

Comparing and analyzing data elements for a particular program or service area could identify program successes, weaknesses, utilization trends, or other budgeting trends of that service or program. For example, comparing pre-established budget thresholds to the number of monthly admissions may help to identify whether the program is successfully meeting its budget. Consider the following scenario: an adult program must maintain an average daily census of 20 patients to be financially stable and 25 patients each day to be financially profitable. When analyzing the data for this program, the analyst identifies 5 of the 31 calendar days in which the program did not hit the 20-patient target. This could indicate a predicated financial downturn in the coming months that will need to be addressed by the management teams. An organization's budget is what drives everything in the organization; therefore, having good, reliable data will assist with the analysis to ensure that the budget numbers are met.

DEFICIENCY

A deficiency is an error found in a medical record that goes against policy. For example, if hospital policy requires every physician order to have a signature, date, and time, then an order with a signature but no date and time would be considered a deficiency. Some deficiencies can be resolved by the HIM staff when they are performing the quantitative analysis. All unresolved deficiencies are carefully logged and tracked for departmental management to review and for notification to the providers. The Joint Commission requires hospitals to perform record analysis in order to identify deficiencies; furthermore, organizations will have policies and procedures related to how long those deficiencies can be outstanding before the physician is held accountable and possibly suspended from certain privileges, such as admitting patients or performing operations.

Deficiency Rate

A deficiency rate is a method of measuring the number of charts with deficiencies found against the total number of discharged patient records for a given period. This calculation and monitoring of the rate is required by the Joint Commission, who require hospitals to have a deficiency rate of no more than 50% of their average monthly discharges. A simple example of a single month's deficient rate could be that ABC Hospital has 250 discharges. Forty of the 250 records contained deficiencies resulting in a preliminary rate of 16% for the month of May 2020. However, the Joint Commission requires that the deficiency rate is calculated using the average monthly discharges of the past 12 months because monthly discharges are ongoing like the timing of when physicians can resolve deficiencies. Because deficiencies are logged into a database or in the EMR, the number of active or unresolved deficiencies can easily be pulled to calculate the deficiency rates.

Data Sampling

Data sampling is a method in which a small selection is analyzed as a representation of the larger whole. For example, a critical care unit has an average of 30 discharges a month. Leadership will pull an audit size of 10 charts to identify the overall representation of all 30 records. If 10 of the records have a similar error, the probability is that the error is present in the remaining 20 records that were not part of the sample. There are two methods of data sampling: random and nonrandom. With random sampling, the data are pulled without guidelines, which will offer a more stratified selection of charts. In a nonrandom sample, the samples are pulled purposefully and target a specific population or trigger. Consider the following examples of data sampling:

- **Nonrandom data sampling**: A manager pulls data on one specific provider who has had a readmission rate of 65%. The manager will only look at that one provider's 500 patient records.
- **Random data sampling**: The manager cannot realistically analyze 500 records; he may only take 10 patient records at random from each month of the study period.

Policies and Procedures for Data Management and Information Governance

Disaster Preparedness

A **disaster** is defined as a catastrophe that drastically hinders the overall functioning of a workflow. Organizational disaster plans will typically address the rollout of the plan when the disaster is apparent, address the dissemination of roles and responsibilities to staff during the disaster, and then they provide recovery measures for when the disaster is over. Disasters should be rated on the likelihood of occurrence and have a specific plan depending on the disaster type. Consider the following scenario: it is more likely that a power outage will occur rather than a flood because a given facility is not geographically located near waterways. Therefore, the HIM director would implement a power outage disaster plan that includes downtime procedures, preparatory training on downtime forms for staff who have only used the EMR, and recovery measures such as back data entry of important data fields that are used for regulatory reporting.

Information Governance (IG)

Information governance (IG) is a set of processes and metrics that is used to ensure that a goal or initiative is achieved. State and federal agencies have data collection requirements that they will analyze in support of their initiatives, and IG will ensure the accessibility, reliability, and transparency of information. For example, suppose state agencies wish to reduce population obesity; they may require healthcare entities to collect and report on patient body mass indexes (BMIs) as a way to measure the progress of the initiative. As another example, a federal agency wants to reduce healthcare costs on co-occurring medical conditions associated with tobacco use. It may require healthcare entities to make referrals to cessation programs to reduce overall tobacco use. IG is important when adjusting processes or workflows to meet requirements because it helps mitigate the predicted crises or shortcomings of an organization's strategic plan.

Data Management and the Challenge of Implementation

Data management is a component of information governance that focuses on specific data elements and their collection. Aspects of data management to be considered are ensuring that the data are reliable, accurate, and transparent. Ensuring that the data being collected meet these criteria can be challenging due to obstructions to the implementation of data management initiatives. Consider the following scenario: to measure outcomes, patients will be asked to fill out a symptom rating questionnaire on admission and another at discharge. The overall management of the data will be easy because it is just the difference between the two scores. However, the staff will now be required to sit with the patient to read or explain the form, which may lead to a decrease in staff productivity. Therefore, weighing whether the data management implementation will be meaningful and beneficial to the patient, or if it will offer no additional benefit to the overall quality of care or services being provided to the patient is essential.

Flowchart

A flowchart is an analytical tool that depicts the steps of a process in a picture format, allowing viewers to easily transition from one step to another step. Flowcharts are often used when outlining the steps in a process, and they are often used as building blocks to drafting policy and procedures. Because the policy and procedure will not always have the inner workings of the actual workflow that staff will encounter, a flowchart can assist with the training and in demonstrating how the process could repeat in some areas. The following flowchart depicts a chart analysis process.

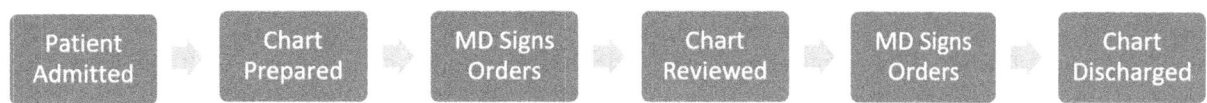

Depicting procedures in a flowchart assists with training new staff and with reeducation needs for current staff; it also assists leadership when identifying areas for improvement.

Turnover Rates and Staff Retention

Staff retention is critical when it comes to reducing turnover rates. High staff turnover can exhaust established staff because it takes time and energy to continually train new staff. When organizations have well-established and -maintained policy and procedures, job aids, and other reference materials, it will help employees to be self-sufficient when questions arise and leadership is unavailable. Although there may be many uncontrollable factors that contribute to turnover rates at a particular facility, ensuring that processes are clearly documented, staff are well trained, and everyone is given access to tools that are designed to help them succeed will help with staff retention. In addition, it is essential to foster a healthy work environment with a focus on improving staff satisfaction, as well as enhancing a culture of respect and trust that the organization and the employees are doing worthwhile work.

Health Record Content and Documentation
Health Record Uniformity

Uniformity in the health record means that there is similarity or consistency across records, forms, charts, and reports. Even though medical record forms may vary from unit to unit or from one specialty to another, there should be uniformity within that same record set. Record uniformity is important for marketing purposes; i.e., the hospital logo on every form makes for a neat and easily identifiable company form. Chart assembly uniformity will assist with orienting readers to the records' structure and provides ease of finding the documents they seek. Uniformity with clinical forms is exceptionally important when it comes to quality-of-care standards, training of staff against company policy and procedures, which often correspond to clinical medical record forms, and assurances that staff are using the forms in the way they were intended. Some uniformity standards and best practices will be derived from governing bodies who define how clinical documentation should be collected and presented.

QUALITATIVE ANALYSIS

Qualitative analysis is the review of a medical record from a quality perspective, in other words, determining if the documentation content thoroughly meets the purpose of the form. Qualitative analysis can be a focused review of a single form or a section of a form, or it can be a full initiative throughout several forms. Consider the following scenario: a patient is admitted to ABC Hospital with suicidality. The admission assessment states that the patient's suicide plan was to overdose on pills. The nursing assessment stated the patient already did overdose on pills, and the psychosocial assessment outlined a completely different suicide plan altogether. This qualitative analysis would result in a low score because it reveals that perhaps staff are not reading and reviewing previously written documentation and are not clarifying details and historical content with the patient. Low qualitative analysis scores may impede the quality of care being given to the patient and could have clinical and administrative consequences.

QUANTITATIVE ANALYSIS AND DELINQUENCIES

Quantitative analysis is the review of a medical record to ensure that the required parts and pieces are present; that all entries are signed, dated, and timed; and that any delinquencies are identified. For example, every obstetrics record will have the same six core documents. A quantitative record analysis ensures that all obstetrics records have those six required documents. Additionally, when ancillary consultations, labs, or other tests are ordered, the quantitative analysis staff person will ensure that the corresponding consultation report and studies are present in the record. This analysis also ensures that all documents and physician order forms are written appropriately and are signed, dated, and timed.

When something is missing from a quantitative review, it is called a **delinquency**. Delinquencies identified during quantitative analysis will be monitored, flagged, and given to the attending physician for correction or clarification. Delinquencies that fall outside the standard are required to be tracked against the facility's monthly discharges.

POOR DOCUMENTATION PRACTICES

The quality, completeness, and reliability of medical record documentation are what define good documentation. Poor documentation falls short of this; for example, physicians may abbreviate words or use unapproved abbreviations. Reducing the use of abbreviations to only approved abbreviations set forth in the organization's policy for the medical record would immediately improve documentation. Poor documentation practices include illegible handwriting, misinterpreted clinical information, and missing or incomplete information. Consider the following scenario: a nurse misreads a medication order as 2.5 mg rather than 0.5 mg, and as a result, administers the wrong medication dosage to the patient. Poor documentation could lead to patient events, negative outcomes, customer complaints, and poor overall quality of care.

FORM DESIGN AND MANAGEMENT

Whether the form being developed is in paper format or in electronic format in the EMR, the form should meet certain criteria—criteria set forth by organizational policy and procedures and regulatory guidelines. In other words, a poorly developed form whose creator did not consult with clinical contributors or regulatory requirements could result in poor patient outcomes.

For instance, suppose a staff nurse fills out a form and reliance upon the information reported in the form resulted in a patient incident. It was identified that the form was filled out incorrectly, and it did not include instructions for how to complete the form. This is an issue that would have been prevented by maintaining an up-to-date form inventory.

Form management ensures that all forms are reviewed and updated routinely. Good form design includes clearly displaying patient identifying information, having proper headings and spacing, and having completion prompts for staff. Forms should be easy to understand by staff of all expertise levels and should serve the required purpose of patient care. A form number or bar code demonstrates that a form has been approved by the appropriate channels and is a key component of form design and management.

Compliance with Uses and Disclosures of PHI

Patient Access to Their Health Information

Authorized Person

Requests for medical records must be pursuant to state and federal guidelines. The Health Insurance Portability and Accountability Act **(HIPAA)** and other state privacy laws require that an **authorized person** can request medical records. An **authorized person** is a person able to act as the patient's representative, e.g., be the adult patient, legal custodian, or a parent of a minor. Stepparents, foster parents, or noncustodial relatives are not authorized persons.

For instance, suppose the HIM department received a medical record request on a deceased patient signed by the patient's brother who claims to be acting on his brother's behalf. In New York State, for example, the only way to obtain medical records is for the executor of the estate signed by the surrogate's court to present paperwork and be the signee on the "authorization for release of information" form. It is important to know state and federal privacy laws that govern access to a record set including mental, public, or medical health records or substance abuse records.

Verification

Verification, or proof, of one's identity can be provided using knowledge of the patient's date of birth, last four digits of a social security number, an address, or even the approximate admission and discharge dates. Another is to compare a signature to the medical record.

For example, a minor patient, who is now an adult, is requesting copies of his medical records. It is unlikely that the requestor's signature will match something that he signed as a minor. Verification is easy when comparing a parent's signature to the minor child's record or even an adult to his or her own record. However, in this case in which the minor has grown to an adult, the HIM department should ask for photo identification along with the signed authorization to match the signatures. In some cases, in lieu of photo identification, one should request a notarized signature affidavit signed by a notary public. Doing this will offer assurances that the person signing is who they say they are.

Minimum Necessary

Although there is no clear definition from the federal register for minimum necessary, HIM and other healthcare-related fields along with HIPAA and other state privacy agencies have recognized **minimum necessary** as being the very minimum access to PHI required to do a job task or to fulfill the intended purpose of an inquiry. Minimum necessary most commonly relates to the disclosure and access to PHI. Consider the following scenario: a patient's elementary school nurse supplies a provider's office with an authorization that requests the "whole record." Unless the school is offering the student a full scope of medical services, it is unlikely that they need the *entire record*. The minimum necessary to provide to the school nurse could be a list of recently prescribed medications, a clinical summary, letters to support nursing interventions at school, and possibly aftercare plans if the student was recently injured or hospitalized. Anything more without an intended purpose would be *more* than the minimum necessary.

ATTENDING PHYSICIAN APPROVAL PROCESS

Though permissible, access to medical record documentation and its contents holds varying levels of risk should the patient gain access to it before a physician has explained its meaning. There are state and federal laws that allow facilities to restrict access in the event it would cause harm to the patient or someone else. For instance, suppose a patient requests a copy of his medical record, which contains abnormal laboratory findings. The patient interprets the lab results as a positive cancer diagnosis and as a result makes life-altering decisions. This is why physician approval is required prior to disclosure of records to the patient. It requires a risk assessment from the physician and in some cases, allows the physician time to reach out to the requestor to ensure that the information will not be harmful to him or her or someone else once known. In some scenarios, the physician can deny access to the medical record based on an increased risk of detrimental harm to the patient or someone else.

PATIENT RIGHT OF AMENDMENT REQUESTS

An **amendment** is one of HIPAA's patient rights when information is being added to the medical record. An amendment is requested to suggest a change to information that the patient feels is erroneous or to add supporting or clarifying documentation to information already in the record. Consider the following scenario: a patient has written an amendment request to clarify that her migraines started at age 23 not age 13, which could be a simple documented edit to the record. Another patient may want to clarify his or her timeline of events of a home incident that they feel is misrepresented in the record. Although an entity cannot deny a patient's request to insert an amendment into the record, every amendment or request for a correction should be appropriately recorded and investigated to identify the legitimacy of the information. Because it is against most state and federal laws to blindly edit, change, or delete clinical information based on an amendment request, it is critical to have appropriate policies in place for record amendments.

OBTAINING HEALTH INFORMATION FOR PATIENTS AND FAMILIES
ACCESS CONTROLS OF DECEASED PATIENT'S RECORDS

In most states' release-of-information laws, a patient advocate or administrator is assigned to take care of a deceased patient's affairs. What is acceptable for banking or educational releases may not be appropriate to gain access to medical or psychiatric medical records. For example, in New York State, once a patient is deceased, the healthcare proxy assignment is no longer valid. The deceased patient's sister requests records from the HIM office in New York State, and she presents the death certificate along with a release signed by the person with power of attorney and an attorney. Unless the individual with power of attorney is named the executor of the estate assigned through the surrogate's court, the request is invalid and insufficient to request medical records. It is critical to understand each state's law surrounding access to deceased patient records because it could result in a lawsuit and violation of access should records be disclosed in error.

ETHICAL ISSUES AND RELEASE OF INFORMATION

When a decision conflicts with a moral standard of society, it is an **ethical issue**. Issues range from staff choosing to misuse PHI for their personal gain, to intentionally omitting or failing to present data accurately to present a better outcome. For instance, suppose a biological father is requesting his daughter's medical record, but he is in prison. This may be perceived as an ethical issue by the staff as to whether he should be receiving records while in prison. However, state and federal laws have outlined who is or is not authorized access to patient information. In this case, regardless of whether the father is incarcerated, he is authorized to access the patient's record. Ethical issues hold risk of noncompliance or legal action. In other words, the biological father could file a complaint and sue the hospital if they refused him access to his child's record. Organizational policy and procedures will address how different scenarios shall be handled and outline laws that should be consulted when ethical issues arise.

REDACTION

Redaction is when a part of or a section of sensitive information is obscured from view or access for legal, security, or training purposes. Redaction is not a deletion or omission of information; it is still obvious to the reader that information exists, but it is censored for the viewer. For example, screenshots used in a training manual have the actual patient's name and date of birth blacked out. It is obvious to the trainee that a true patient name is present, but for privacy and security reasons, the trainee can't read what the patient's name is. Similarly, an optometrist may request medical records from a hospital; however, the patient did not authorize the release of HIV information. Because HIV information has special protections, staff will be required to redact that information from the record before releasing it to the optometrist. Redaction not only protects the information of the patient; it also protects the interests of the organization by maintaining compliance with various laws.

INCOMPETENCY OF A PATIENT

HIM offices may receive inquiries of information from the parents of adult children. Although an individual older than 18 or 19 years may rely on his or her parents, they are still considered an adult under the law and are required to make decisions. When validating a request for an adult patient signed by his or her parent, it is important to inquire about the patient's ability to sign or make healthcare decisions. **Incompetency** is typically court ordered and is when a person has been deemed unable to make healthcare decisions. Like a power of attorney, a person is assigned as a primary caregiver of that adult. For release-of-information purposes, the document signed by a judge deeming the patient to be incompetent is required for record disclosure. Consider the following scenario: the father of an autistic adult patient wishes to assist him in obtaining copies of his medical record. The HIM department will inquire about the patient's ability to sign the authorization form himself. Once told that the patient is incompetent, the HIM staff should request the court order as supporting documentation to validate and authorize the disclosure of the records.

OBTAINING PHI FOR AN ADOPTED OR FOSTERED PATIENT

A **foster parent** is an adult caregiver who is assigned by county services to temporarily care for the well-being of a minor. In this case, the county maintains custody of the minor. An **adopted parent** means that the parent went through the court system to obtain legal parental rights of a minor and, for all intents and purposes under the law, has the same rights as a biological parent. It is critical to understand the custodial status of a minor patient when disclosing medical records because custodial parents have healthcare decision-making rights. For instance, suppose an HIM office receives an authorization signed by a foster mother. Because the foster mother does not hold custodial rights, the authorization should be signed by the county services designee. Whereas, if the same authorization is signed by the adopted mother, access is warranted under the law. Though disclosure of PHI is of a low risk when it pertains to coordination of care and treatment efforts, it can hold some risk of complaints or litigation when disclosures are made pursuant to an unauthorized individual.

Legal and Regulatory Standards for Healthcare Information Requests
Health Record Types and Disclosures of PHI

The record keeping of a specific subset or specialty of services in which an entity provides is called **health record types,** and the components and organization of the record will be unique to that health record type. Types of healthcare records could include:

- Medical or physical
- Psychiatric, behavioral, or other mental health
- Substance use or abuse treatment
- HIV, genetic testing, or health data related to research studies
- Long-term care

Equally important is how the record is maintained and disclosed. Protocols and requirements for this are derived from state and federal standards. Consider the following scenario: a patient's signed HIPAA authorization form may allow the disclosure of medical information, but that same form may not contain the language needed to legally disclose HIV information. Therefore, it would be against the law for the entity to release HIV information should it be documented in the record. To comply with the law, the HIV information would need to be redacted prior to being disclosed. Alternatively, staff would need to obtain a properly signed authorization that allows the release of the HIV information. The same actions would apply for any of the above protected record types.

Subpoena Duces Tecum, Court Order, and So-Ordered Subpoena

Subpoena duces tecum is Latin for "you shall bring with you" meaning a legal request to bring relevant documentation with you to a court hearing. Subpoenas are typically signed by attorneys. A **court order** is the same request for relevant documentation only if it is signed by a judge of the court, and a **so-ordered subpoena** will be signed by an attorney and a judge of the court. It is important to understand which document above is required to disclose certain record types. For example, in New York State, a court order or so-ordered subpoena is required to disclose mental health records. If a subpoena duces tecum is received, it is invalid until a patient-signed authorization accompanies it. Some state laws outline the disclosure of certain record types and whether they should be shared in open court. Therefore, disclosure of records pursuant to one of the above legal requests, along with the proper disclaimer required under the law pertaining to an "in a judge's chambers" record review or an open court review are critical.

Law Enforcement Requests for Information

Law enforcement is considered any person or entity that has been given the power to enforce the law including, but not limited to, city police officers, county sheriffs, officers of the court, and officers of various state or federal agencies. It is important to know that the HIPAA Privacy Rule still applies even when law enforcement is requesting PHI. Patient authorization is almost always required to disclose PHI to law enforcement. Under certain circumstances, limited demographic or nonspecific patient conditions could be released in the event that a criminal case is being investigated. For instance, suppose a police officer calls the operator of a local hospital inquiring if John Smith, a missing person, is there receiving treatment. The operator cannot confirm or deny whether the patient is currently an active patient. On the other hand, if a properly identified police officer inquires whether John Smith is an active patient because John Smith is the subject of a criminal investigation, then the entity can disclose limited demographic information and dates of service. Anything pertaining to the patient's health, psychiatric, or other medical condition is prohibited without patient authorization.

Release of Information in Relation to Treatment, Payment, and Healthcare Operations

TPO, or treatment, payment, and healthcare operations, is outlined in HIPAA as permissible circumstances to use or disclose PHI without patient authorization:

- **Treatment** could indicate any kind of continuity-of-care efforts, emergency room or crisis center interventions, or off-site physician practices that also hold privileges at the local hospital.
- **Payment** could indicate internal or external record audits for the entity to receive payment for services rendered. At times, federal or private payers will require documentation to support that services were provided and for which they received bills.
- **Healthcare operations** could indicate any internal uses of PHI such as using patient records to conduct audits and to perform internal investigations, case studies, training and education, and other activities unrelated to direct patient care.

Although TPO uses and disclosures are permissible, some entities have policies in place to still require patient authorization for certain circumstances. These are usually related to PHI with special protections such as HIV, mental health, and substance use.

Privilege

Privilege relates to the relationship between a patient, his or her provider, and the confidentiality of information documented in the medical record. Privilege belongs to the patient, not the provider; in other words, the patient expects the physician to maintain the confidentiality of his or her health information. Access to such information is protected under HIPAA as well as other state and federal laws. When medical records are requested as part of litigation, or when a patient's provider is being called as a witness in court, it is often required that privilege be waived, meaning the patient has signed a consent form that allows his or her information to be shared. In other words, the permission by the patient or authorized person is granted to breach that confidentiality for the purpose of the legal matter. Consider the following scenario: a psychiatrist is subpoenaed to testify in court. Privilege must be waived for the medical doctor to speak in court about the patient's confidential information. Privilege can be waived via a signed authorization for records or written permission by the patient for the psychiatrist to testify in court.

PHI within the Organization
Record Access Auditing

Federal regulations require monitoring of record access to ensure that the privacy, confidentiality, and integrity of a patient's medical records remains intact. As such, it is important to have thorough access audits and knowledgeable staff analyzing the reports.

For instance, suppose a recent access audit revealed that a staff member was accessing a patient's record who the staff member was not actively treating. In this scenario, it is imperative to reconcile whether the access was appropriate or not. Access to medical records is permissible only when there is a need to know the patient's information to do a job duty. Identifying access of staff not on the treatment team violates company policy but does not necessarily mean that the access is malicious, and it may or may not be a breach of patient privacy.

Begin by identifying which screens the user viewed. Determine if the user edited, viewed, printed, deleted, or created a document or information. Pull the access audit from different avenues to view access in different ways. Aspects to consider are the duration of the access and whether a previous or subsequent patient had a similar name, date of birth, or MRN. Reconciling this information will help in the investigation of whether the access was inadvertent, malicious, or done out of curiosity.

HIGH-PROFILE-PATIENT ACCESS

High-profile patients are those who meet certain criteria that increases the scrutiny of how their PHI is handled, maintained, or accessed. Examples of high-profile patients include a renowned community socialite receiving treatment at a rehab or the victim of a severe car accident whose accident is in the daily newspaper headlines. These events hold significant risk for inappropriate access by staff due to the publicity surrounding the person or event. High-profile-patient policy and procedures should be developed to ensure that the patient's privacy is maintained. It should include how staff access the records, how and when the record is then locked down from the general staff population, and how it is audited and used in the future. Consider the following scenario: hospital leadership uses a high-profile patient as a case sample in a staff meeting. Although all records should be held to the same privacy and access security standards, due to their greater risk, the use of high-profile patients or events, even within the organization, should be limited.

ACCESS MONITORING WITHIN AN ORGANIZATION

Access monitoring is a security measure that ensures that staff, students, interns, or others with PHI access are in fact accessing that PHI appropriately and within their job scope. It is critical for those monitoring staff access to be informed when staff float to other clinical areas; are promoted, demoted, fired; or have otherwise had their access or scope of practice changed. Knowing this information will improve the quality, accuracy, and legitimacy of the access audits. Other access monitoring considerations consist of knowing whether the entity has ancillary or off-site locations, whether the EMR is a shared system or a stand-alone system, and defining what would constitute inappropriate access as defined by federal laws.

NEED-TO-KNOW PRINCIPLE

The **need-to-know** principle in HIM is a component of the minimum necessary requirement. In other words, determine whether staff *need to know* the specific information to complete a job function. This may mean that certain staff need to know some but not all of the information to do their job. For instance, a patient accounts person does not need to know the clinical picture of the patient to perform his or her job duties. Therefore, it is reasonable to have security measures in place to prevent patient accounts staff access to the clinical portions of the medical record.

The need-to-know principle should be considered whenever patient health information is being accessed. It is sometimes subjective and relies on the decision making of the staff person, and sometimes it is restricted by federal or state regulation. The need-to-know principle should also be applied when reviewing security access to PHI, disclosing PHI, and sharing PHI while the patient may be actively receiving treatment.

AUDIT TRAIL

An audit trail is a recorded series of computer events that traces user activity. All events on an audit trail are dated and time stamped. A typical audit trail will include when a user logs into the operating system or application and what activity was performed such as adding, removing, deleting, moving, editing, printing, viewing, or accessing screens within that environment. Audit trails are used to prove or disprove the appropriateness of business activity, access to PHI, or legal matters that occur in the computer system. For example, a hospital could print out the audit trail of an employee to prove that the employee did not intentionally delete files.

Retention and Destruction Policies for Healthcare Information

Record Retention Policies and Guidelines

Record retention is the duration or length of time that records should be maintained. The term record includes medical records, business records, operating or financial records, patient account records, human resources or payroll records, environmental reviews, and more. Records created to operate or maintain business information are important to that business for various reasons, and, as such, the proper keeping and archiving of those records are essential.

Both federal and state governing bodies outline regulation about record retention. Although it's customary to maintain most business records for only 7–10 years, some obstetrical, gynecological, newborn, and deceased-patient records are kept for a much longer period of time. It is important to understand what is considered part of the legal medical record and what are considered to be business documents of your organization. Once clarified, identify which state and federal agencies monitor, audit, license, or accredit such documents or programs correlated to the documents. It is considered best practice to retain records for the longest period or most stringent rule outlined by state and federal agencies.

Certificate of Destruction

A certificate of destruction is required by HIPAA after the disposal and destruction of patient health information. These certificates are required as proof that PHI was destroyed according to HIPAA guidelines. They document who did the destruction, when and what was destroyed, how the information was destroyed, and any witnesses to the destruction. If outsourcing the destruction of PHI, organizations must ensure that their business associates have proper certificates of destruction. According to the US Department of Health and Human Services (HHS), who enforce HIPAA, PHI should be disposed of by shredding, burning, pulping, or pulverizing so that the PHI is unreadable, undecipherable, and cannot be reconstructed.

Proper Destruction of PHI

The destruction of medical records is most often thought of to be in the form of shredding. To that end, when shredding highly confidential information such as medical records, HIPAA guidelines require a P-3 shredder, or a shredder that cross cuts the paper into strips of certain lengths and widths to eliminate the risk of reassembly. However, when considering the destruction of PHI, it is important to note that PHI can also be used and stored on CDs, DVDs, microfilm, x-ray film, or other media. The protocols for the destruction of those media must also ensure that they cannot be reconstructed or deciphered in a logical way. Consider an information technology (IT) specialist who has been asked to dispose of an out-of-date fax machine. Because the machine holds memory, albeit limited, one could use the machine to recreate and print any stored data from a previous faxing process. To properly dispose of the machine, the IT specialist should destroy the memory card first.

Record Retention Monitoring Efforts

Record retention is an archival practice of maintaining and retaining records in an off-site location for an extended and defined period. The length of time that record types should be retained is defined by state and federal statutes. Archiving records for too short a period of time will lead to noncompliance under some laws, and too long of a retention could result in a breach of PHI compliance. Consider the following scenario: an HIM staff member identified a box in off-site storage that contains records from 30 years ago. The staff member steals some of the PHI for malicious purposes. The facility would be at fault because that box of records was long past the legal retention requirements, putting the information at risk. Identifying what pieces of information should be archived off site and defining the retention schedule for that information will assist in properly maintaining the integrity of the record keeping and access process.

Record Retention and the Budgetary Process

Retaining boxes of either medical or business records can be costly. A best practice has historically been to box records and send them to an off-site location for its retention cycle. Budgetary implications associated with a physical retention center will be the monthly or annual rent for storage as well as environmental controls and access fees associated with retrieving records back to the facility for various purposes. Comparing such retention efforts and costs to converting to a digital solution could be beneficial. The cost of digital storage as opposed to physical storage could be drastically cheaper. In one hypothetical case, suppose that rather than boxing the monthly hall checks, the unit clerk scans them into a shared folder on the computer. The staffing and supply costs associated with scanning the volumes of information to be retained could in the end be equal to or exceed what physical storage would cost. Thus, it is important to understand what needs to be stored and for how long before outlining costs associated with any storage solution because it will have budgetary implications.

Release-of-Information Workflows

Decreasing Turnaround Times

The **turnaround time** is the difference between the start date and the completion date of a given project, initiative, or workflow. For example, a request for records that was received on June 1 was processed and mailed on June 7. The turnaround time is 6 days. Expected minimum turnaround times are set by regulatory bodies; in other words, the state licensing agency requires that records be processed within 10 days. Other times (either averaged or maximum times) will reflect best practices or policies set forth by the organization. When the actual turnaround time exceeds the expected times, leadership will break down the workflow, observe staff performing their functions, and monitor their productivity reports. In addition to these steps, calculating average turnaround times and graphing them over time will assist in identifying trends. This information is crucial to the process of decreasing turnaround times because the trends can highlight steps in the process that are consistently struggling.

Requestor Type

Requestor type is the entity or person(s) requesting PHI including, but not limited to, outpatient providers, attorneys, schools, and county social workers. Understanding who is asking for patient information and the frequency at which it is requested can help streamline release-of-information workflows. Consider the following example: county child protective services workers frequently request the same five data elements with every request. This could be an opportunity to create a standardized form to meet their needs on an ongoing basis without having to release multiple pages of a patient's record. Other requestors could be an outpatient provider who is a frequent referral source for the hospital or the local school district with an on-site medical clinic. Release-of-information tasks could be streamlined, and the number of PHI requests could be drastically reduced if those specific requestor types are given contractual access to the EMR, so they can pull clinical information as needed on mutual patients.

Clinical Summary Versus Record Copies

Although the most accessible and frequently disclosed format is an actual photocopy of the medical record, access to PHI does not always need to mean a photocopy. A **clinical summary** is a brief narrative describing the overall clinical picture of the patient and their treatment at a facility. For instance, suppose a psychiatrist wrote a six-page progress note outlining in detail the past and present social, family, and educational status of their patient. The patient's college has requested the "last progress note" to assess the patient's need for educational assistance. Rather than provide the school with the actual last progress note in its entirety, the psychiatrist chose to write a clinical summary in its place. The summary would outline the reason for treatment, the prognosis, and the strengths and weakness that could be addressed by the school. The clinical summary would leave out explicit patient details in order to meet the minimum necessary standards while still protecting the remaining content of the clinical medical record.

Benefits of Tracking ROI Workflows Electronically

Tracking when a request for information is received, when it was fulfilled, and what PHI was disclosed to whom is required under state and federal laws. For example, John Smith requested his record on October 6; on October 9, Mary, the clerk, mailed the five-page discharge summary from the patient's August inpatient stay. Identifying these elements for one patient is easy because the request and its disclosure information is found with only that one patient's chart. However, when large amounts of data are requested to identify trends and other ROI statistics, having the ROI workflow information stored electronically will assist with the data-gathering process. When ROI workflow data are stored electronically, accessing the data for analyzing turnaround times, staff productivity, and the frequency and volume of request types becomes easily accessible. It can also streamline invoicing, reduce other costs associated with record copies, and prioritize work distribution among staff.

Trust-But-Verify Principles

When staff are professionally trained, there is a reasonable expectation that they can work independently without constant supervision. As it relates to release of information, which is a high-risk area due to the sensitivity of the information, the staff should be trained in and held accountable for proper handling of that information. The number of requests of a facility can be overwhelming, and it is unrealistic that a supervisor will double-check the staff's work before or after it is processed. **Trust but verify** is a principle that enables staff to work freely under the direction of a supervisor. The supervisor trusts that the employees are performing the task correctly and periodically verifies that this is true. Ways to foster a trust-and-verify workflow include spot checking completed tasks against the policy and procedure, cross training staff on different job tasks, encouraging questions, and, when necessary, assigning riskier tasks to more experienced staff.

Breach-of-Information Protocols
Parties to Notify

According to HHS, breach notification must occur without unreasonable delay and no later than 60 days after the breach is identified. Furthermore, when a breach occurs and is identified, the following entities should be notified under certain circumstances:

- The individual whose information was impacted
- The media and other local news outlets when 500 or more individuals' information is impacted
- The secretary of HHS, either annually when fewer than 500 individuals are impacted, or no later than 60 days when more than 500 individuals are impacted
- Some states require breach notification to the state attorney general and other entities.

It is critical to be sure that the organization's breach notification policy and processes are up to date and that staff is trained to ensure timely notification.

Violation vs. Breach

According to HHS, a **violation** is a failure to comply with the privacy rules and regulations outlined in the law. A violation can be one of malicious intent, such as unauthorized access to PHI, or it may occur inadvertently, such as a staff member photographing her office space forgetting that PHI is visible in the photo. A **breach** is a HIPAA violation in which an impermissible use or disclosure, as defined under the HIPAA Privacy Rule, compromises the security or privacy of PHI. In other words, the difference between the two is that when PHI is compromised and it causes financial or emotional harm to the patient as a result, it is categorized as a breach. For example, if a person hacks into the hospital EMR and steals PHI for financial gain, it would be considered a breach. HIPAA violations and breaches can hold heavy consequences for the staff member and for the entity. Penalties can be of a monetary or litigious nature or may potentially include prison time. As such, it is critical to have extensive training and monitoring programs in place.

Breach Investigation Response Process

Once a breach is identified, it is critical to begin the investigation process because there are specific time constraints regarding notification. First, leadership should take immediate actions to stop the breach. Contact the privacy officer who will commence the formal investigation and have a full understanding of the timing of the breach notification steps. The privacy officer will work to identify where, when, and how the breach occurred and collaborate with other leadership to mitigate the effects and correct the breach. Human resources should be involved early in the process should sanctions or other disciplinary actions be required due to the breach. Lastly, it is critical to identify if the breach is reportable to the patient, secretary of HHS, and other outlets under HHS guidelines. Most investigations will result in findings or conclusions with recommended action items. Those action items should be implemented without delay to reduce the likelihood of the event repeating.

PHI Breach Prevention Measures

Risk mitigation and prevention are the best methods to protect against a breach occurrence. Risk assessments should be conducted annually to identify threats and vulnerable areas in staff training and education of HIPAA standards; to access controls and monitoring; to ensure that administrative, physical, and technical safeguards are developed and implemented; and to encourage a positive culture of reporting without repercussions. Consider the following scenario: two staff members discuss their previous evenings at home. One discloses that they lost the patient file they brought home to work on. In that moment, the other staff member should be reporting the breach to leadership; however, in a culture of nonreporting, there is a fear that the other party will also get in trouble if it is reported. Ensuring that all staff are trained on HIPAA-related policy and procedures, the appropriateness of handling and monitoring PHI, and the safety of reporting noncompliance are all critical in reducing the risk of breaches.

Breach Notification Letter

The breach notification rule requires that when a breach has occurred, and under specified circumstances, the entity must make certain notifications. One of those notifications is to the individual or source patient of whose information was breached. For example, Mary Jones' medical records were stolen out of storage and later found in a dumpster. Mary Jones must be notified of the breach because it was her PHI that was violated. A breach notification letter should be sent to the individual without unreasonable delay, no later than 60 days after discovery, and requires the following specific elements:

- A brief description of the breach and the circumstance that led to the breach
- The type of parts of the patient health information that was compromised. For example, the name, date of birth, social security number, or clinical information such as diagnoses, etc.
- Steps that the individual should take to reduce the risk of harm because of the breach; for example, if he or she should monitor their credit report or call their providers or family to seek emotional support
- A description of the steps that the organization will or did take to mitigate the breach from reoccurring
- A facility contact person as well as an HHS contact number if the person has concerns or complaints about the breach

COMPLIANCE WITH PRIVACY INITIATIVES
ADMINISTRATIVE SAFEGUARDS

The HIPAA Security Rule's largest component is the requirements under the administrative safeguards. The administrative safeguards rule itself is categorized into several sections, some of which include security management and incident management, staff education and in-services, workforce access and development, and the implementation of business associate agreements. Successful administrative safeguards will be comprised of thorough and routinely reviewed and updated policy and procedures, access and security risk assessments, identification of vulnerabilities and other risk areas, contingency plans, supervision and termination plans of staff, and staff training needs. Consider the following vulnerability: a hospital does not discuss HIPAA at a new employee's orientation and, as a result, the new staff member publicizes patient information on social media. The administrative safeguards are required to ensure that the fundamental activities and practices within the organization are compliant with patient confidentiality and privacy laws.

PHYSICAL SAFEGUARDS

Physical safeguards are a set of policies and procedures set forth by an organization that ensure that PHI is protected from natural or other environmental conditions that could be considered destructive to PHI, such as flooding or fire, as well as protection from unauthorized access. Policies and procedures related to disaster preparedness are critical to keeping PHI protected under the physical safeguard rule. Physical safeguards include the following:

- Sprinkler systems are in place.
- Doors are kept locked with one-way access.
- PHI is kept out of public view.
- Printers, fax machines, and shredding bins are strategically placed.
- There is a limited assignment of office keys.

The HIPAA Security Rule requires entities to have physical safeguards in place and to ensure that the staff is educated and knowledgeable about those safeguards.

TECHNICAL SAFEGUARDS

Technical safeguards are required under the HIPAA Security Rule. These safeguards consist of the overall technology of how PHI is used and accessed in the EMR or ancillary systems that use or maintain PHI. Consider the following vulnerability: a hospital assigns the same password to all new staff and does not require it to be changed upon first log in. In time, a staff member has gained access to unauthorized areas of the EMR due to this gap in the password policy and practices.

There are various ways that technical safeguards can be implemented that will protect PHI from unauthorized access. IT departments will develop and use popular security rules such as user-based and role-based assignments for staff access. **Role-based** access would consist of all nurses having the same computer access, whereas **user-based** access would separate one nurse from another nurse based on what each nurse's specific job tasks are. Additionally, there is context-based access, emergency access when PHI is locked, transmission security, access control, and audit controls, all of which are critical when developing technical safeguards.

Patients' Rights Under HIPAA Related to Access Restrictions

One of the HIPAA patient rights is the patient's **right to access**. In other words, the patient can request, under reasonable conditions, access to their medical record. For example, John Smith calls the HIM department to request copies of his entire medical record. Under the HIPAA law, the HIM department cannot deny the patient access to his record. There are other recourses to be taken in the event that the information could be harmful, but the information remains John Smith's, and his access is permitted under the law. Routinely, to meet a request such as this, providing the patient with a physical photocopy of the record will suffice. However, if the information could be harmful, an appointment could be made with the physician or designee, so that the patient can gain access to the information while having someone available who can answer any questions related to the information.

Patients' Rights Under HIPAA Related to Confidential Communication

Confidential communication is a HIPAA patient right. This means that the patient can request that staff contact them at a specific phone number only, or, while in public spaces, he or she can request that staff move to a private location to discuss PHI. Consider the following scenario: Suzy has requested confidential communications and for staff to only call her cell phone number; therefore, if a staff member called Suzy at her home number or contacted her via her email address instead, then it would be a HIPAA violation and a possible patient complaint. It is important to have strong policies and procedures in place to ensure that staff are well trained on how to recognize when patients have requested a specific means of confidential communication.

Compliance with Security Initiatives
Data Encryption

Data encryption is a method in which the true data are hidden or displayed into another format until the recipient has the code or key to appropriately access the materials. Data encryption is often used when transmitting PHI through electronic means to maintain the integrity and confidentiality of the information being transmitted; it reduces the risk of unauthorized access. There are three common types of data encryption:

- The **Data Encryption Standard (DES)** is a 56-bit level of encryption and is no longer considered to be a safe encryption method given its size limitations.
- The **Advanced Encryption Standard (AES)** is a 128- to 256-bit level of encryption that is standardized into today's facilities that use highly personal and sensitive information.
- The **Rivest–Shamir–Adleman (RSA)** encryption algorithm helps with the transmission of data between two locations. With RSA encryption, a public key encrypts the data whereas a private key is used to decrypt the information.

Security Threats

A security threat is any vulnerability found in technology, devices, hardware, or the overall infrastructure of an organization that allows PHI to become vulnerable to unauthorized access. It is impossible to prevent all security threats because technology is always advancing, as are the methods by which criminals seek to gain unauthorized access to PHI and hospital systems. HIPAA requires that entities perform risk assessments to not only identify the vulnerable areas in their technology but also to identify preventative measures and the likelihood of a threat being successful. Proactive and preventative actions should then be taken to reduce the risk of a security threat.

Remote Desktop Method

A remote desktop is a security safeguard that IT departments use to maintain access control over their systems and programs. The use of a remote desktop also eases the burden for IT to install updates, apply patches, and add or remove programs for widespread use. Furthermore, it allows the flexibility for staff to work from home because all users are accessing the one terminal server on the entity's grounds or in one secured location. Consider a hospital with 500 staff members all needing access to the same programs. Rather than IT having to apply system updates to 500 unique desktop computers, the update would only be applied to the one terminal server because all 500 staff members access the hospital programs through the remote desktop.

Two-Factor Authentication

Two-factor authentication is a security safeguard and method of access control to a secure application or operating system. Two-factor authentication requires at least two pieces of criteria that ensure that the person requesting access is who they say they are and has authorization to access the application or system. Authentication is usually confirmed using a physical feature, information known only to the person, or an item given to the person such as a radio-frequency identification (RFID) tag or keycard that is interfaced with the security access controls. Consider the following scenario: in order to log in to the EMR system, a staff member is asked for a username and password along with a six-digit code. The code is generated by a token, given as part of the onboarding process, which displays a new code every 25 seconds. The strength of this safeguard lies in the fact that the chances of an unauthorized person being able to successfully determine more than one of these criteria on their own is extremely low.

E-Signatures

An e-signature is a method of authentication that allows someone to sign their name via a computer or other electronic means, rather than with pen and paper. It is common to have a method of authentication to ensure one's identity prior to applying an e-signature. Various state agencies have a policy in place that allows for e-signatures. For example, the New York State Electronic Signatures and Records Act signed into law that electronic signatures are as legally binding as handwritten signatures, as well as how they should be formatted. A handwritten signature is considered a **wet signature**. Someone could "sign" their name on an electronic pad and have it mirror their handwritten signature on the electronic form. Another method would be a digital format with the words "electronically signed by" and a date and time. Laws would require that entities who adopt e-signatures have proper authentication policies and procedures in place. Forms that do not have the standardized statement with the date and time would indicate a lack of proper verification and authentication practices.

ORGANIZATIONAL COMPLIANCE WITH HEALTH LAWS, REGULATIONS, OR STANDARDS
MOCK SURVEY

A mock survey is a simulation of a true regulatory survey. It is essentially a practice run that mirrors survey activities and examines the facility's readiness for the actual regulatory survey without consequences. Mock surveys are usually conducted through a third party and, as such, are a paid service. Consider the following example: two individuals present to the reception desk and announce that they are from the Joint Commission. The mock survey in this case is focused on whether the staff at the desk know the next steps that need to take place. Also, during a mock survey, the two individuals who are pretending to work for the Joint Commission will also assist, train, and advise the staff and leadership on how to increase their readiness for an actual survey. Mock surveyors will give consultative feedback, which will assist the facility in making improvements where needed to prepare for a better outcome during the actual survey. Mock surveys should be conducted prior to an actual survey and with enough time to initiate changes where recommended.

ROUNDING

Rounding is like a mock survey only on a much smaller scale. It typically occurs frequently to ensure ongoing compliance and understanding with facility policies and procedures, regulations, laws, and standards from accrediting or licensing entities. Rounding can be done by facility leadership rather than a third party. For instance, suppose the HIM director rounds on the patient care units to be sure that PHI is inaccessible to the public; he or she will also inquire with patient care staff about common HIPAA principles. Staff training needs or other corrective actions identified during rounding activities should be identified quickly and closely monitored until correction or reeducation occurs. Doing so will increase the staff's readiness, familiarity, knowledge base, and comfort level for when state and federal surveyors do present at the facility.

PATIENT TRACER

A patient tracer is an auditor who follows the clinical path that a patient took while in the hospital using only the documentation in the medical record. A patient tracer is one of many preparation methods aimed at mirroring survey activities and helping to review regulatory licensing or accrediting compliance. Consider the following example: the HIM director pulled a discharged patient's chart. As the director reads through the chart, he would present to each service area and review that area's documentation as well as inquire with staff about other regulatory compliance measures. This tracer activity could result in identifying documentation that could be misleading, unclear, incomplete, or noncompliant with the standards. In other words, a patient transition from one service area to another was not clearly documented in the record. Patient tracers can also help identify staffing re-education needs and areas in which the quality or continuation of care or how patients are using services throughout the hospital can be improved.

ONGOING POLICY AND PROCEDURE REVIEWS

A **policy** is the outline of principles and reasons of why a task or workflow should be done. Policies are derived by governing bodies, and when they are not followed, it could result in consequences. **Procedures** are the clearly defined and documented steps taken to execute the policy successfully. Policies and procedures are developed for clerical workflows, nursing interventions, or other organizational activities that need to be carefully followed. For example, suppose a patient incident occurred in 2020 because of an incorrect nursing intervention. The staff nurse on duty was trained on policies and procedures from 2015 when she started employment. The corresponding policies and procedures hadn't been updated and were out of date. Regular reviews of policies and procedures are imperative when it relates to direct patient care, regulatory workflows, or frequently updated practices in health care. Staff should be trained against them and have access to all policies and procedures that relate to their job functions. Staff should also be re-educated whenever a policy or procedure is updated.

CORPORATE COMPLIANCE COMMITTEE

A compliance committee is an interdisciplinary group of individuals in an organization who meet periodically to ensure that the organization remains compliant with state and federal regulatory bodies as well as the licensing, accrediting, and certifying bodies for the organization. The role of the compliance committee includes the following:

- Review a summary of facility HIPAA breaches
- Review customer complaints along with investigative outcomes
- Monitor the successful rollout of risk assessments
- Carry out action items identified from systemic areas of concern
- Conduct audits that relate to the reimbursement practices of the facility
- Ensure that human resource practices are complaint and fair to all staff

The committee is typically formed to ensure that all aspects of the entity are compliant with all governing bodies to which the entity would need to report.

Data Analytics and Informatics

PRODUCTIVITY REPORTS

STANDARDS AND REPORTING OF STAFF PRODUCTIVITY

Productivity standards are measurements that define how something should be output. Productivity standards are usually derived from best practices and shorten the learning curve when it comes to training on-the-job tasks. Implemented productivity standards ensure that workflows are successful, that staff are held to the same benchmarks as their peers, and that job tasks are completed in a uniform way.

A **productivity report** is a display or summary of outputs against the standard. Consider the following scenario: the productivity standard for record analysis is 10 charts per hour. An HIM staff member is analyzing 12 charts per hour. The individual is a high producer and ensures a successful workflow. Another staff member analyzes 4 charts per hour, which is a low performance rate against the standard. Productivity reports should be run over a period of time to identify if the staff's compliance is ongoing or is an isolated occurrence. Productivity should also be compared to staff quality reports to ensure the overall success of standards.

USE OF PRODUCTIVITY REPORTS IN DISCIPLINARY PROCESS

Running staff productivity reports and comparing them against the productivity standard can assist with promotional opportunities; identify process, training, or PIs; or even establish grounds for disciplinary action or termination when the productivity reports are chronically low. Consider the following scenario: for six months, leadership has monitored the productivity of a staff member. The staff member's productivity report continues to show low performance even after relocating the staff member's desk, purchasing an ergonomic chair, and re-educating the staff member on job aids, as well as the related policies and procedures. When a staff member is consistently falling below the productivity standard on an assigned task, it could mean that he or she needs additional training or other supports to improve productivity, especially when peers are meeting or exceeding the productivity standard for the same task. In extreme cases, low productivity scores on a report could indicate that the staff member is no longer qualified for the job at hand.

BENCHMARKING

Benchmarking is a full analysis of data or results and comparing it against the data or results of the same standard either internal or external to the organization. For example, a 200-bed medical hospital compares its readmission rates to similar hospitals across the US. A benchmark is a target based on that comparable data. Inconsistent or unrealistic expectations, outcomes, or targets are at risk of being set if that organization compares their data to those of organizations different from themselves. Using the example above, the 200-bed medical hospital would not want to benchmark their readmission data against a small 80-bed rehabilitation facility because the size of the facility and the specialties are different. A rehabilitation facility may have a higher readmission rate solely on the nature of the conditions that it is treating. Benchmarking is important for organizational quality programs because the aggregated data are used to determine if quality indicators and expectations are being met.

CROSS TRAINING

Cross training is a practice in which a person is trained in more than one skill or job task in a department. The benefits of cross training can include the following:

- improved department agility
- improved staff flexibility
- reduced need for outsourcing
- reduced feelings of staff being overwhelmed or overworked
- increased staff motivation and collaboration
- improved departmental or staff longevity
- improved productivity, efficiency, and turnaround times

Consider the following scenario: an HIM department's turnaround times for processing records were high and resulted in low productivity for the coding and billing staff. Then, three of the HIM clerks receive cross training on record prepping, quality control, and record analysis. As a result, the HIM staff can now process 10 times as many records in an hour because they have the fundamental knowledge of all three jobs, can work more efficiently, and can jump into any of those roles should the need arise. If more staff have been trained on a given task, it increases the flexibility and efficiency in how that job is done.

BOTTLENECK

From an HIM perspective, a **bottleneck** is a distinct slowing or blocking of productivity in a workflow. A bottleneck can be a manual or a systematic problem. A manual bottleneck is when the workflow is inhibited directly by an individual. This could be a situation in which a staff member, recently transferred from another station, was not trained properly and, as a result, is not confident in his or her work and performs the assigned duties much more slowly than other staff members. A systematic bottleneck can occur due to broken equipment, connectivity issues, or a lack of staffing. For example, if the scanner stops functioning at the record-scanning desk, then record processing will slow or stop until the scanner is fixed, decreasing the expected productivity. Reducing or eliminating bottlenecks in an HIM workplace is critical for an HIM supervisor because much of what the HIM department does causally relates to the success of patient accounts, coding and reimbursements, and patient care.

SUPPORTING END USERS IN EHR APPLICATIONS
TOOLS AND RESOURCES

Job aids or end-user training guides will be created for step-by-step instruction on how to do a given job task. During an EMR implementation, user guides will not only explain the screens and the screens' purposes, they will also outline the functionality and interaction with other screens or fields in the EMR. Quick guides are intended for immediate reference for staff inquiries and can be presented as cheat sheets, question-and-answer lists, flowcharts, or check lists. A test environment will allow staff to practice real-life scenarios related to their job functions as well as increase the staff's familiarity with the EMR and its overall functionality. It is beneficial for end users to be able to access either EMR superusers or technical staff for allotting time to practice in the test environment and have the opportunity to ask questions. The overall success of an EMR implementation will be determined by the tools and resources given to prepare and support end users during their training.

Test Environment

A test environment is a mirror image of a live patient database. Patient personal information is deidentified, but the clinical data, scenarios, and studies are real. The test environment is used when testing and validating the build of clinical screens when the EMR is being designed. The intention of the test environment is to practice data entry and validate how data feed from specific screens to other areas of the EMR. Testers will attempt to make intentional errors or deletions to validate the functionality of the EMR design. For example, suppose the HIM director enters vital signs into the clinical record. Then a progress note is started, and he notices that the vital signs being pulled into the note are last year's vitals, not the ones he just entered. This reveals an error in the design and functionality of the EMR. Test environments allow these practice runs to fail without putting real patient data or patient care at risk.

End-User Expectations

An EMR implementation is the process in which an electronic record is built and rolled out for end-user activity. There are several stages to an EMR implementation and various starting points at which organizations may begin. For example, Hospital A may implement an EMR from an all-paper record whereas Hospital B may be implementing from a hybrid record, meaning a partially electronic record. At the start of an EMR implementation, the staff should be trained on the use and functionality of the system and its relation to their specific job duties. They should receive training materials such as user guides or cheat sheets as well as a test environment in order to increase their comfort level with the new EMR. By the end and after an implementation, when fully rolled out, staff should expect the EMR to follow their workflow and not the other way around. Therefore, it is critical that those training the staff are clear and thorough when preparing end users. If the workflow is changing from their current routines, it is important to encourage flexibility and willingness to adopt change.

Help Desk Support

A **help desk** is a person or group assigned to assisting the staff of an organization with technology and software needs. They are often responsible for end user and password set up to new applications as well as installing new applications or resetting passwords. A designated help desk can be beneficial and can add value to an organization because it centralizes and maintains control and security safeguards as they relate to security settings and access to PHI. Help desk staff will often have a healthy understanding of all applications used within an organization and how those applications interface with each other. A help desk will assist with early detection of any technological issues that may become widespread as well as notifying staff when systems are or will be down.

Superuser in EMR Implementation

A **superuser** is a high-performing staff member who has been selected for a leadership role during an EMR implementation. The superuser will be assigned to assist with workflow development, test pilot preliminary designs of the new EMR, and train end users. Consider the following scenario: Sarah has been a unit clerk for 5 years, and prior to that she was in medical records for 10 years. Given her longevity and knowledge of organizational workflows, she was selected to be a superuser for the clerical staff. She will be involved in different aspects of the EMR implementation, receiving training opportunities first, so that she will be prepared and available to assist end users during their training periods. Having superusers is beneficial and useful during an EMR implementation because it delegates tasks from other members of leadership and increases the access of knowledgeable people to the end user during training and throughout normal business operations.

Visual Representations of Data for Decision Making

Analytical Tools in Relation to HIM

Analytical tools are instruments or visual depictions of data that assist in the decision-making process. Analytic tools could be considered graphs, charts, or diagrams that are created to review a significant amount of data in a simplified picture from different business, clinical, or financial perspectives. Using analytical tools will often answer descriptive or predictive questions such as why or how something is happening, when something may happen, and steps needed to prevent something from happening. Histograms, pie charts, bar graphs, and line graphs will offer visual displays of data and will quickly and easily identify trends and tell the data's story. A **fishbone diagram**, or a cause-and-effect diagram, is another visual aid when investigating the root cause of a specific problem or crisis. A pros and cons chart may help in the decision-making process when suggesting new contracts, vendors, staffing, or business needs.

Impact of Trend Line on Decision-Making Process

A trend line is a line on a graph that shows the general direction or course that something is taking. For example, on a graph depicting an organization's monthly discharges, the trendline is dipping to the right. This would indicate that the trend of monthly discharges is decreasing. A trendline that is dipping to the left would indicate an increasing trend. Noting how a trend line behaves over time can help to identify areas of healthy performance or areas that need improvement. Consider the following two graphs representing no-show rates. When looking at the monthly no-show rates of a medical practice, the trend line reveals an increase in no shows over time. This would initiate change. However, when looking at the same no-show data weekly rather than monthly, the trend line may falsely show that the trend of no shows is decreasing or staying the same.

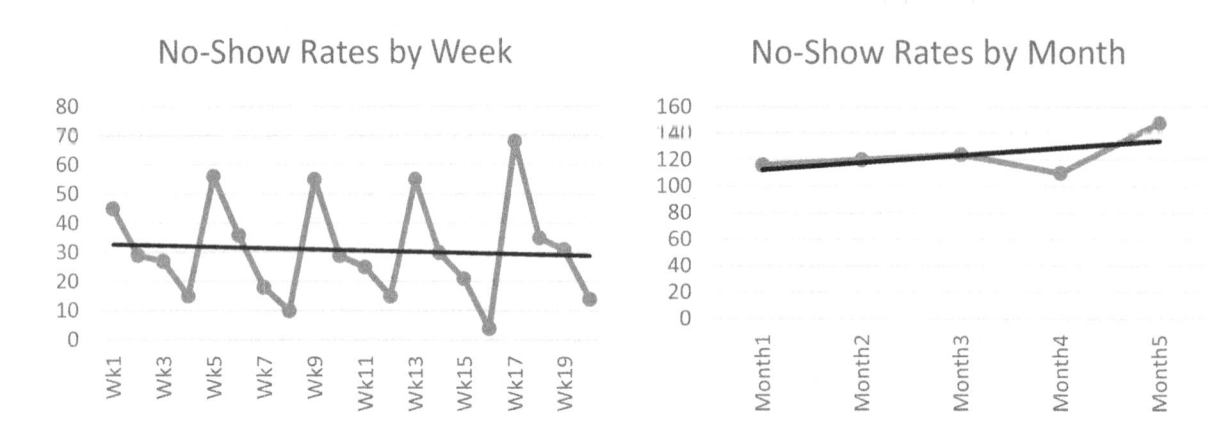

It is important to identify what the standard should be for an indicator and then measure rates consistently over time; that way, the data suggest a more accurate trend line.

Root-Cause Analysis

Root-cause analysis (RCA) is a methodical review of a specific problem or incident with the goal of identifying the event that caused it. An RCA is typically required by state or accrediting agencies when a significant incident occurs or a series of similar incidents. This could be triggered by a single patient death or by noting a pattern of several patient injuries in a short amount of time. An RCA subcommittee is formed of several disciplines; each will review a copy of the investigative materials such as the medical records, staff and patient interview notes, photography, and relevant policies and procedures. The subcommittee will then discuss and determine the following:

- Causes of the problem
- Solutions to the problem
- Ways to enact the solutions
- Measures to assess the effectiveness of the proposed solutions

SENTINEL EVENT

A sentinel event in health care is defined by the Joint Commission as any unanticipated event in a healthcare setting that results in death or serious physical or psychological injury that is not related to the natural course of the patient's illness. In other words, if a patient is admitted to a hospital for a hairline fracture in their femur but ends up passing away, it would be classified as a sentinel event, because a hairline fracture does not routinely result in death. Other examples of sentinel events could be patient falls, an object left inside a patient after an operation, or even an operation being performed on the wrong body part. Sentinel events must be thoroughly investigated and are typically subjected to a full RCA. Tracking and monitoring sentinel events will allow healthcare organizations to review their patient care practices, policy, and procedures; improve quality of care; and help prevent those events from occurring in the future.

FISHBONE DIAGRAM

A fishbone diagram is an analytical cause-and-effect tool that depicts potential problems in specified areas. A fishbone diagram is often used during an RCA or other investigative reviews. Taking into consideration and outlining the contributing factors during an investigative analysis will help identify the roots of an incident in such a way as to illuminate how it should be corrected and prevented from happening again. The factors that make up the bones of the fish are as follows: measurements, materials, personnel, environment, methods, and machines or other technologies. The problem is outlined in the head of the fish. Identifying failures in any of these contributing factors could lead the investigator to the conclusion that there is a single problem or several problems and room for improvements. Once these are identified, actions must be taken to prevent future occurrences. Below is an outline of a fishbone diagram.

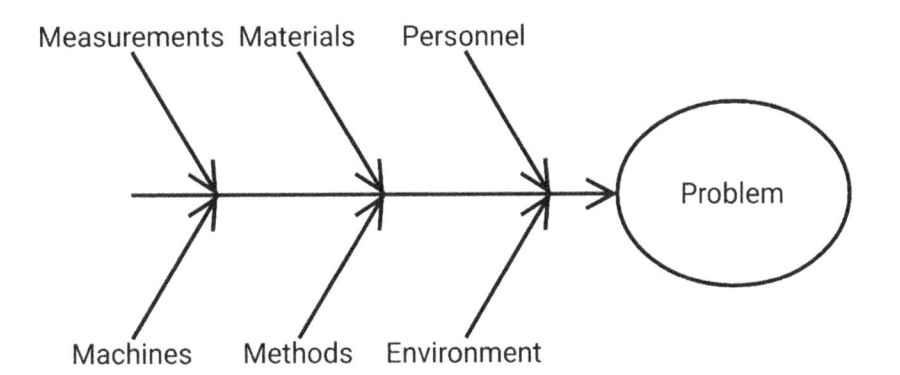

SUMMARY REPORTS BASED ON TRENDS

COLLATED DATA RESULTS

To collate data means to collect and organize them in a unified order. Collated data summaries highlight trends and overall findings of the data either in monthly or quarterly report mechanisms. When reviewing cases individually, it may be unclear if the findings are widespread or isolated events. A monthly or quarterly summary will collate all of the findings into digestible categories. Consider the following scenario: an analyst discovered 10 findings surrounding record completion. Each of the 10 had a different example of an omission. It would be too cumbersome for the analyst to share each individual finding with management because it would not display the same level of significance as collectively saying, 10 out of 100 charts for the month of June had omissions. Decision makers cannot make organization-wide decisions when the data are too fragmented and difficult to review.

STEERING COMMITTEE

A steering committee is a subset group of a larger group made up of different disciplines who are the primary decision makers and developers of an anticipated initiative. If ABC Hospital wants to purchase and implement a medical record scanning solution, then a steering committee may consist of the following members:

- The HIM director for HIM expertise
- An accounting department member to help analyze the costs associated with the project and budget appropriately
- An IT designee to assist with reviewing the specifications of the equipment, storage capabilities, and interface functionality
- Someone from the clinical staff may also be included to help identify which parts of the medical record would be beneficial in the scanning solution and which pieces should remain in other formats.

It is essential to have committee members with various expertise and knowledge assist with the implementation and ensure that the overall goals of the project are met.

COMPARING MONTHLY AND YEAR-TO-DATE DATA

It is routine for HIM departments to collect and report on monthly or quarterly statistics. An example of a monthly statistic may be a measurement of the number of admissions and out of those admissions how many had a history and physical (H&P) completed within 24 hours of admission, which is a Joint Commission standard. If the monthly result is reported without comparing it to the year-to-date number, it will become difficult to identify if a noncompliance issue is isolated to one month or if it is widespread over time. An ongoing comparison of monthly and year-to-date data could also assist with identifying annual situational circumstances. For example, in the month of July every year admissions drop; however, by November the year-to-date numbers are meeting budget expectations. Consider the following chart, which will outline how one month could be an outlier but the year-to-date number remains within the target.

	Month	Year to Date
Admissions	35	412
H&P on time	22	380
% H&P on time	63%	92%

USE OF HEALTHCARE STATISTICS

Healthcare statistics are collected in order to measure the success of patient outcomes, quality initiatives, and the overall financial successes of business. For example, nursing leadership may measure and use statistics based on staff incidents such as needle sticks or nursing turnover rates. Physician leadership may measure mortality rates, medication errors, or utilization of services statistics. Specialty services such as cardiology may measure more specific data such as mortality rates due to cardiovascular disease compared to myocardial infarction. The administration may look at statistics based on the number of patients that are served in the various areas of the hospital and compare those against the budget numbers. Other statistics would relate to regulatory measures such as timeliness of documentation or percentages of compliance on quality standards. Examining several different healthcare statistics will offer evidence of effective services and patient care, as well as performance and financial successes or weaknesses.

Upper and Lower Control Limits

Upper and lower control limits are statistical boundaries depicted on a graph to identify whether the data are accurate and comparable to the other data points being displayed. The upper limit is the highest value allowed for a data point before it becomes a statistical outlier, with the lower limit being the lowest value for a data point before it is a statistical outlier. The upper limit is calculated by adding the mean and the standard deviation of a data set. The lower limit is calculated by subtracting the mean and the standard deviation of the same data set. The graph below shows how eight data points fall within the upper and lower control limits, one point falling below the lower limit and one point falling much higher than the upper limit. This data point should stand out as a statistical anomaly and should be investigated to determine what caused it.

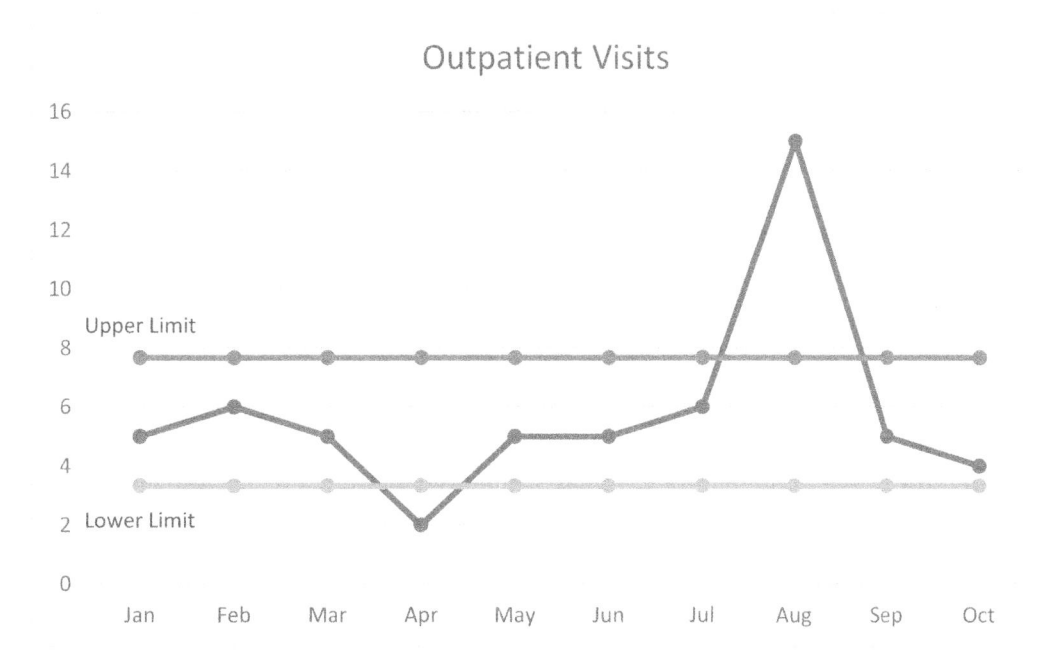

Database Management Techniques
Metadata

Metadata are essentially data about other data. Metadata are collected, indexed, and stored in the system background. For example, suppose an HIM clerk scans a lab result into the medical record. To the viewer, only the lab result that the clerk scanned would be visible. However, the metadata collected would consist of the user ID of that unit clerk as well as the date, time, and procedure code that was saved into the system memory. Metadata are collected on every piece of data activity that takes place in the system. If data are entered, deleted, edited, moved, or altered in any way, metadata are collected on that activity. Metadata are considered business documentation as opposed to patient clinical information and are discoverable under litigation should allegations of fraud be presented. If metadata are collected on each system activity, it would be impossible to hide fraudulent activities.

Data Warehouse

When multiple systems send data into a single location or repository to be collated and used for multiple purposes, this repository is called a **data warehouse**. Data warehouses are used and maintained for several purposes including the following:

- immediate delivery of PHI for patient care use
- data reporting to identify trends or other analysis
- to centralize all data in order to monitor and maintain data integrity
- freedom from source system limitations

In other words, data warehouses ensure complete reporting and output capabilities, whereas some of the source systems, pharmacy, or laboratory systems, for example, may be limited in reporting capabilities. Metadata are analyzed and monitored in "data marts," or miniature data warehouses, for system specific discrepancies before being delivered to larger data warehouses.

Structured Query Language (SQL)

Structured Query Language (SQL) is a programming language that is used to build most databases. SQL can be used to store, retrieve, delete, or edit information. SQL is based on relationships between data points offering methods to organize and structure the data so they can be used later. The query is a way for the data to be reported based on given criteria. In other words, a query is a question about a large amount of data that will then be structured in a way to answer that question. SQL can be complex; therefore, knowledge of computer coding principles and understanding how the data relate to one another is needed in order to create databases, queries, and reports. Fluency in SQL aids in understanding end-user needs and expectations, which will help drive the initial development of the database. Knowledge of SQL is critical for data engineers, front- and back-end database programmers, and mobile application developers.

Importance of End-User Analysis to Database Management Techniques

Understanding end-user needs and expectations is critical for database management because it lays down the foundation of the database. Suppose Tom, a database engineer, creates a database to collect restraint and seclusion data for a psychiatric hospital. He failed to ask and learn that the end user wanted to measure the average days between the patient's admission and the first restraint or seclusion event. Now this measurement cannot be collected because the database was not designed to include the date of admission. To have a successful database, one needs to have reliable data, be able to identify users who need and want to use the data, and have the knowledge base to develop a user-friendly system. An inability to understand or neglecting to inquire about end-user needs or expected uses of the database will ultimately result in a poorly developed, insufficient system that could unnecessarily cost the organization extra time and money.

Redundancy in Database Management

Redundancy is an occurrence of duplication in a system or a subset of data. For example, an EMR requests that the vital signs are entered in three different locations. Redundancy can put patient care or other patient care activities at risk because of erroneous data entry; in other words, one vital sign location may read differently than another causing an error in clinical decision making. In this vital sign example, this redundancy can be eliminated if the nurse enters the vitals into one location and the other two locations pull the data from the source location. Querying databases for duplication errors as well as monitoring them for redundancy issues will assist with improving patient care outcomes and improve the use of and the outcome of the data being gathered. Eliminating redundancy in an EMR or any database is critical when identifying whether that redundancy will have patient care, financial, or other organizational implications.

Master Patient Index (MPI)
Documenting a Patient's Alias Name

An **alias** is when a patient identifies by a name other than their legal name. For example, Frederick, who likes to be called Fred at work, goes by an alias of David Jones when he travels for leisure. If David Jones is the name of a real person who also lives in the same geographic area as Frederick, there is a chance that their medical records could become compromised or mistaken for one another's. An alias could also be the maiden name of a married person, the birth name of an adopted child, or a new legal name given to a patient who now identifies as the opposite gender. When discovered, documenting the alias of a patient can assist in continuity of patient care, reconciling loose reports when filing in the medical record, and/or identification of the patient years later in the master patient index (MPI) should the patient return to the facility seeking care.

Monitoring MPI Quality

The **master patient index** (MPI) is a library of all patients who have received services at a facility. The index is often maintained and updated by the HIM department. Key elements of an MPI, at a minimum, are the patient's name, date of birth, alias, admission and discharge dates, and sometimes diagnoses. Because patients will often seek services more than once in their lifetime, it is critical to have trained staff monitor and maintain the integrity of the MPI. Poor maintenance of an MPI could result in the loss of records, an increase in MRN duplication, or over- or under-disclosure of PHI. For instance, suppose a patient received treatment at a facility three times before marriage and once more after she was married. When asked for records, the HIM department only released the first three episodes because the MPI did not present the fourth admission—because it was under her married name, was given a new MRN, and was separated from the other records.

Sunsetting of an EMR

When an EMR "sunsets," it means that the vendor has announced a future date in which the program will no longer be supported. With an unsupported EMR, a healthcare facility cannot continue to document and use the EMR with assurances that the information will be properly maintained and that the core functionality of the program will continue to work the same way. When vendors sunset a program, it is critical for facilities to seek out and implement a new program. Once selected, it is possible to have existing patient admission, discharge, and transfer information migrate to the new program. However, the quality and success of that migration depend on the upkeep and quality of the MPI. Any misspellings, missing data, typos in dates or names, duplications, or other errors will then be migrated to the new program as true source data. It is critical to have knowledgeable and trained staff maintain the MPI to ensure its high quality and to ensure the integrity of the data.

Duplicate Medical Record

A duplicate medical record is when two or more MRNs are assigned to the same patient. This unintentional discrepancy causes the medical record information to become fragmented, inhibiting the ability of the physician to see the full clinical history and picture of the patient. It is critical that staff who are professionally trained and are attentive to detail be responsible for reconciling MRNs. Patients often have the same names, same dates of birth, or same addresses over time; however, they may not indeed be the same person, or on the contrary they are indeed the same person. Consider the following scenario: a duplicate MRN report identifies John Jones with a date of birth of June 6, 1956, and John Jones with a date of birth of June 6, 1965. At first glance it would appear to be two different patients 9 years apart in age; however, a closer look at the record identifies this as a simple typo. When two MRNs are assigned to the same patient, a merge can be performed. A

merge will consolidate the PHI into and under a single MRN. The other MRN would be saved as an alias and cannot be reused for any other patient.

Manual Review Prior to Merging MRNs

A manual review is when staff intervenes with an automated process. Automated reports are great when streamlining workflows; however, a manual review of the data can find outliers that would otherwise be missed. Consider the following scenario: the daily duplicate medical record report suggests that two MRNs should be merged. However, upon a manual review before merging the two numbers, the staff identify that the MRNs belong to a set of minor twins. They have the same dates of birth, same address, same last name, and same phone number. The system automatically used preestablished criteria to determine a likeness between two patients; however, the manual review identified that the first names are one character off, they each have different middle initials, and, additionally, one of the twins has a chronic medical condition whereas the other does not. Confusing medical record information because of a duplicate MRN can have no effect on a patient, whereas other instances can be detrimental.

Audit Documentation Using a Focused Tool
Concurrent Chart Reviews

A concurrent analysis or chart review is when a record is reviewed simultaneously to when the patient is receiving treatment. Concurrent chart reviews could be disruptive to the workflows being conducted because the reviewer must review live and in process documentation. Reviewing the record concurrently is beneficial because it allows time to identify and correct findings that may have become out of compliance with regulatory standards or a negative patient event. Consider the following example: an HIM staff member presents on the unit with a concurrent analysis checklist in which she must review the following: data labels on every form; physician orders containing a signature, date, and time; the absence of blanks throughout the forms currently in the record; and any documents such as the H&P, which is required within the first 24 hours of a patient admission. This checklist tool would review completion, uniformity, and accuracy and would be used to do a concurrent review because it would immediately identify problem areas early and offer time for correction.

Retrospective Chart Reviews

A retrospective chart review is looking back after something occurred. In other words, reviewing a record after the patient has completed or is discharged from receiving treatment. A retrospective chart review is often triggered by a complaint, questionable practices, or findings during a concurrent audit. Its results will identify findings, practices, or trends that occurred in the past and over time. From a process improvement perspective, retrospective reviews can also be used to compare to concurrent reviews to see where PI initiatives have strengthened or weakened. Consider the following examples: a concurrent audit identified an untimely H&P examination. An HIM clerk performs a retrospective review on the timeliness of the H&Ps over the past 3 years to determine if this has been an ongoing discrepancy. In another scenario, the risk management department received a complaint about Dr. Jones, and the pharmacy technician is asked to perform a retrospective audit on medication-prescribing practices that would then be compared to medication-prescribing best practices.

Performance Standards

Performance standards are a set of expectations or a list of requirements predefined and approved by management used to evaluate staff and quantify how well they are doing in their jobs. Performance standards can be job specific and based on productivity expectations or can be related to professionalism, customer relations, bedside manner, phone etiquette, etc. Suppose Sam received her annual performance review and scored low on the professionalism standard due to the six customer complaints she received in the past year, which exceeded the performance standard of no more than two customer concerns in a year. Because Sam had more than the allowed amount, she scored low in the performance standard. Consistently scoring low in one or more standards could be grounds for disciplinary action.

Audit Consistency

An audit can focus on record completion, quality, comparison, investigative, financial, or other measurements to obtain a needed outcome. Regardless of the purpose of the audit, it is critical to have consistency. Although there will be variation in the sample pulled to be sure that the full scope of the inquiry is audited, it is important to use the same audit tool across the whole sample. For instance, suppose Luis audits 10 records for discharge summary compliance and notices that Dr. Jones has not been compliant. Because Dr. Jones is his favorite doctor, Luis skips the compliance questions and uses a different tool for Dr. Jones to hide the noncompliance with discharge summaries. Audit consistency will ensure that there was no favoritism, oversights when auditing for specifics, or allegations of fraud. All documenters will be held to the same requirements and standards when their records are being audited using the same audit tool or other measurements.

Takeback and Reimbursement Audit

Reimbursement audits are exceptionally important for hospitals to consider due to the potential of takebacks from state and federal payers. Monetary **takebacks** occur when payers identify that reimbursements were made for services that were not accurately billed, rendered, or documented appropriately. These audits are retrospective, meaning that the payers will review records on services that they have already paid to ensure that the reimbursement was appropriate. A takeback may not impact large organizations, but for small organizations it can be crippling. HIM departments should collaborate with accounting or patient account departments to conduct regular reimbursement audits. These audits sample charges over a whole month and identify whether the corresponding physician orders, progress notes, group notes, or other documentation requirements exist to support the bills. Doing this proactively will greatly reduce the risk of a successful takeback by a payer.

Health IT to Improve Workflow

Abstraction of Patient Information

Abstraction is the process of retrieving data from a source document or field and placing them in an automated system used for data analysis. Abstraction can be cumbersome when manual intervention is required to pull information from paper or electronic records. However, abstracting data from an electronic source is fast and easy when it relates to pulling large amounts of data. For example, management wants to pull BMIs on 300 patients. This is a relatively simple process because the information is stored electronically in a data field in the EMR. Once the BMIs are pulled out of the EMR, the data are processed by another system that will quickly analyze and summarize them. Abstraction can be a useful tool when completing data entry for regulatory core measures or when meeting organizational goals or other regulatory needs. If the data are in a data field or check box in the EMR, then those pieces of information can be abstracted and loaded into the core measuring system directly, which will drastically reduce the manual data entry efforts and time.

Scanners

Using scanners in an HIM department has many benefits. It can reduce workflow turnaround time, improve productivity, save on manual data entry efforts, and save space in the office by reducing the need for shelving and cabinets. Scanned documents also allow for easier access to PHI by more than one caregiver at a time. Because there are several scanning solutions to compare when considering one, it is important to understand what will be scanned and how frequently information will be scanned. A single-doc scanner is beneficial to a front desk clerk who has one or two documents to scan. Single-doc scanners are compact and only handle one page at a time. Batch scanners are used when scanning multiple patients' documentation or a batch of forms at one time. Batch scanners are larger and work best when forms are bar coded. Barcoded forms assist with the indexing of the document, whereas a single-doc scanner may require manual indexing.

Unconventional Uses of an EMR

Non-EMR, or paper record, environments relied on knowledgeable and educated staff, whereas with the development of EMRs many of those tips, hints, and education points are built into the EMR. For example, in a paper record a nurse may have used a printed drug–drug interaction table; however, with an EMR, the system will notify her of an interaction systematically. A well-developed and well-used EMR will not only be used for patient care but also streamline many other healthcare functions and operations. For small office practices, an EMR will streamline the check-in and check-out processes, speed up scheduling activities, and monitor and maintain physician schedules. An EMR can also be used as a scanning solution, a repository for reporting patient incidents, risk management, and release of information. Most EMRs also have the capability for billing activities as well as administrative functionality. From another patient care perspective, EMRs have the capability to interface with pharmacy systems, which will then automate the drug interaction risks as well as allergies or observation statuses that are red flagged and could cause harm to the patient.

Encoder

Often interfaced with the EMR, an **encoder** is software used to enhance coding practices from a diagnostic and procedural perspective. In other words, the encoder will read material in the medical record to assist in assigning diagnostic or procedure codes. An encoder can be logic based, prompting the coder to answer specific questions, and then it assigns codes based on the coder's responses. Although an automated codebook format resembles a physical codebook, the software makes the reference search, code identification, and code assignment much easier for the coder. As such, encoders increase the productivity of coders, which in turn results in the success of the revenue cycle, and an encoder often maintains up-to-date coding guidelines to ensure the overall quality and accuracy of coded records.

Interface

An interface is a connection or region between two different computer systems that share and exchange data; in other words, it is a bridge from one computer program to another program. For instance, if a hospital has an interface between the EMR and the pharmacy system and a patient is admitted, discharged, or transferred between units, then that information is automatically updated in the pharmacy system. Interfaces will often be created to streamline duplicate data entry, ease manual staff interventions within workflows, and improve the quality of documentation and patient care because the opportunity for errors is drastically reduced. Because interfaces can be costly to an organization, it is critical to ensure that the interface serves a significantly beneficial function to the organization. The success of an interface lies with its purpose, how it is built, and in ensuring that the fields from one system match the data structure of the other system.

Health Information Exchange (HIE) Solutions

A health information exchange (HIE) is essentially a large medical record repository for a large geographic area. An HIE for a state is an EMR to a local hospital. For example, the New York State HIE is called "Hixny," or the Health Information Exchange of New York. It's a data repository to which smaller EMRs, entities, organizations, and provider offices belong and interface their PHI data with. An HIE is generally used for the coordination and collaboration of care. Suppose Dave is on vacation 6 hours from home. He needs medical attention but is not a good historian given his condition. If access is granted, the emergency room physician could access the HIE in order to review PHI from any of Dave's primary care providers. The more entities that belong to an HIE, the more robust the PHI library, and this in turn increases the availability for other treaters.

An HIE can be used for large data collection for reporting purposes, identifying trends in a population, or providing a historical footprint for patients who are unable to provide or recall critical medical information. An HIE offers a significant amount of history and data, like a patient's medications, laboratory radiology, demographic information, and hospitalization records. Suppose a patient was involved in a motor vehicle accident. She is unconscious and unable to share with the physician that she is anemic. By accessing an HIE in this situation, the patient's medical history would be made available to the physician so she could be treated accordingly. An HIE improves the overall quality and safety of patient care and, at times, the speed in which patients can be treated, which can help reduce organizational costs.

HIE Consent Model

State HIE consent models may vary slightly, but, overall, the consent remains with the patient and is generally an "opt-in" or an "opt-out" model. Contradictory to HIPAA in which the patient consents to the disclosure or use of PHI, in a HIE, the PHI is already sent via an interface and stored in the HIE under contractual agreements between the HIE and the patient care provider. Patient consent does not initiate an entity "sending" their PHI to the HIE because it's already there. The patient consent is initiated at each patient care site, and the patient consents to whether that patient care site may access their PHI from other facilities in the HIE. For example, two local hospitals are members of the HIE and send their PHI as defined under contractual agreements. A patient visits their pulmonologist and signs a consent form indicating that their pulmonologist's office can access the HIE, understanding that the HIE will have information in it from the two local hospitals.

Breaking the Glass

"Breaking the glass" is a patient care activity in an HIE that will allow authorized users access to PHI that they have not yet been granted access to. During the patient consent activity, a patient allows or disallows a provider to gain access to their PHI in an HIE. If the patient did not grant access or has yet to consent to access at a facility, under certain circumstances a provider can break the glass, forcing access to the patient's PHI. Suppose a patient presents to an emergency room unconscious and hemorrhaging. The emergency room physician may break the glass of the HIE in order to identify what medications are prescribed to this patient, any recent lab results that could indicate a hindrance in blood clotting, or even to identify next of kin or other emergency contacts. Because patient privacy and confidentiality laws still apply, all events of breaking the glass are monitored and audited to ensure that the access was warranted and was done appropriately.

Patient's Involvement in an HIE

Healthcare entities are not the only source for HIEs. Patients, parents, and other patient advocates are importance sources when it comes to maintaining the integrity of the HIE. Because HIEs are sourced through local EMRs, most organizational EMRs have implemented patient portals. Some HIEs even have a patient portal that allows the patient or advocate to log in and add, edit, update, monitor, collect, or validate their PHI. Although not all HIEs will offer such specific business activities through their portal, they may offer superficial details such as diagnoses, locations, and recent dates of treatment.

Clinical, Administrative, and Specialty Service Applications

Key Administrative Responsibilities

Hospital activities reach far beyond the patient care activities that are crucial to healthcare operations. Administrative responsibilities are to support activities that help the functionality of healthcare operations. Without administrative functions, patient care initiatives could not be executed. Key administrative functions of any healthcare organization relate to operations, finances, legal issues, communications, and human resources. All of these key functions support the overall clinical and patient care initiatives of the organization's vision. They often do not need direct patient care or patient data in order to function.

Interfaces

An interface is a bridge from one system to another that allows for the transmission of data. For example, a laboratory system can be interfaced with an EMR so that the two systems share the patient name, date of admission, date of discharge, and other relevant data. Interfaces are beneficial in that they reduce or eliminate the need for manual data entry. An interface reduces the risk of duplication or errors in a patient's demographic information and improves efficiency in workflows. Interfaces are often built where workflows or initiatives need to be streamlined. However, one potential downfall to interfaces is if an error occurs in the source data, then those erroneous data will be transmitted to all other systems interfaced with them.

Content Integrity

Content integrity is the validity of information that is collected and displayed for a larger purpose or use. Because administrative activities support day-to-day operations clerically and financially, it is critical that their unique operating systems have reliable, accurate, and dependable data, and that they ensure that the data are content-specific enough to meet their needs. Suppose that the human resources system has functionality that will identify which staff work on which units of a hospital. However, it is not monitored or updated with staff turnovers, terminations, or when life events occur, resulting in inaccurate staffing and communication. Identifying which specific content and data elements should be collected in each administrative system being used will help identify how the integrity of the data will be monitored. Without that content integrity, organizational business decisions will not be made using accurate and reliable data, which could cause time and monetary consequences.

Benefits of Policy and Procedure Application

Stand-alone policy and procedure applications offer one location for all staff members to reference any applicable policies and procedures they need to do their jobs. All policies can be maintained through their editing and approval processes, thus saving policy versioning directly inside the applications. When inquiring about applications that specialize in policy and procedures, it may be helpful to identify if the application has training and development functionality, which will assist in human resource requirements. Additionally, state, federal, or accrediting agencies such as the Joint Commission will interface their standards and regulations with the policy and procedure application.

Benefits of Human Resource Application

An organizational stand-alone human resource application allows HR personnel to monitor staff assignments, time, attendance, training, development, and disciplinary actions among other aspects. Although human resource applications have no need for patient care access or interfaces, the monitoring of staff who are taking care of patients is critical and, as a result, is indirectly related to patient care. If human resources personnel have a difficult time monitoring staff, the organization could be vulnerable to poor hiring practices; high turnover rates; insufficient disciplinary practices; and loss of money related to vacation, sick time, holiday pay, and other staff benefits. Because the Joint Commission has standards dedicated solely to human resources, having a stand-alone HR application greatly improves the success of compliance with the standards.

Healthcare Statistics for Organizational Stakeholders

Discrepancies in Statistics

A **discrepancy** is an inconsistency in data findings. For instance, suppose a renal program met budget numbers for five out of six months, and the sixth month came in dramatically above budget. The spike is unlikely because the renal program can only offer so many services per month. Therefore, the spike is misrepresenting billed services. If not validated, the spike could falsely represent an increase in revenue for that month. Because data are used to compile an analysis of the larger picture and to make financial or clinical patient care decisions, it is critical to ensure that the data are correct. Reconciling any discrepancy in the data results will enable more accurate decision making.

Organizational Governing Body

A **governing body** is a group of people, stakeholders, employees, or community leaders that ensures that the policies and functioning of the organization are being fulfilled properly. Most members of a governing body are voluntary and have a moral and ethical responsibility to the success of the organization. As defined by the governing body, annual, quarterly, or monthly reports of statistical, clinical, and quality data are presented to ensure they are kept abreast of the overall functionality of the organization. Governing bodies review and approve annual budget plans to ensure that money and revenue are being spent appropriately and remain in the spirit of the organization's mission and values.

Impact of Healthcare Statistics on Organizations

Many organizational decisions are derived from healthcare statistics, so it is critical to ensure that the statistical numbers and their analyses are meaningful. For example, a readmission rate for one month is reported as 12.5%. However, there are no other data points to help indicate if this is a high or a low percentage. Therefore, comparing these results to benchmarked results will only be beneficial once a facility understands their statistical relevance. Monthly or quarterly statistics help when analyzing and monitoring the overall functioning of the organization, including individual programs and satellite facilities. Comparing and displaying organization data over time, graphing data against similar hospital's or program's benchmarked data, or even using cumulative averages rather than a simple average are strategic ways of using statistics to ensure that the best decisions are derived from the data.

Cumulative Average

A cumulative average takes the average over a period and bringing it forward to subsequent time periods. This differs from an average, where it is just the average of data for that single point in time. Consider the following scenario: an HIM director reports on record completion statistics. Her current report states the following:

- Records completed within 30 days of discharge = 10%
- Records completed after 30 days of discharge = 90%

Although improvement should be made to increase the number of charts being completed within 30 days, it is the second statistic that is misrepresented. At first glance, it appears that 90%, usually a positive result, of records are completed after 30 days, which could force the assumption that they are completed at 31 days or 35 days. However, the reality is that a record could be incomplete 120 days after discharge but still fall into the 90% because it is "after 30 days of discharge." A clearer way to display these data is through a cumulative average, as follows:

- Records completed within 30 days of discharge = 10%
- Records completed within 60 days = 10%
- Records completed within 90 days = 25%
- Records completed within 120 days = 55%

HEALTHCARE STAKEHOLDERS

A **stakeholder** is someone with a vested interest in the overall performance and success of something. At times, a stakeholder is someone who invested time or money into a business and is waiting for a monetary return on that investment. In health care, stakeholders are other entities or persons who have an interest or concern in the success of the healthcare organization. Stakeholders could be patients, physicians, employees, pharmacy or pharmaceutical firms, healthcare payers, and other insurance agencies because they all have a vested interested in the success of the entity. If the entity succeeds, then the stakeholder succeeds.

Revenue Management

Educating Providers on Value-Based Care Programs and Guidelines
Value-Based Care and Fee-for-Service Reimbursement

In recent years, private and federal initiatives have increased the discussion of value-based programs rather than a fee-for-service-based reimbursement system. Facilities are increasing their patient outcome and satisfaction comparative data to ensure that value-based reimbursements will be profitable. **Fee-for-service** reimbursement is paid out for services individually. In other words, it costs $1,000 for a single laboratory test. This results in increasing the number of services being provided to maximize its probability. The downfall to fee-for-service is that quantity outweighs quality. On the opposite side, the most recent drive for reimbursement change is value-based. **Value-based** reimburses for services based on the patient's outcome and the overall quality of care being provided. Care providers must take the time and meet quality indicators to be reimbursed for services rendered.

Value-Based Care Reimbursement

Value-based-care reimbursement focuses on the quality of care and attempts to reduce the increasing healthcare costs for the patient and the organization. According to the American Medical Association, there are ways to increase the overall quality of care being given to the patient that will set the organization up for success under value-based reimbursement models:

- Patient-centered care, ensuring that patients are active participants
- Leadership and professionalism of healthcare workers
- A robust and reliable IT infrastructure
- Broad access to PHI, which could be achieved through HIEs
- Leadership visions that encourage quality of care and balancing that quality with the quantity or volume of needed services to meet budgetary requirements

Because organizations specialize and treat a variety of conditions, providing specialized or unique services or procedures, there are value-based models that can be contractual to ensure that the organization is getting the most reimbursement for their services and quality that they are providing.

Impact of Value-Based Care on Patient Populations

The fundamental ideal of value-based care is to impact and improve the populations that the organizations serve. The hospital should not only be providing high-quality care, but it should also be encouraging preventative care in order to lower costs for patients and their families as well as increasing patient satisfaction rates, which will, in turn, be marketing and referral sources. In the long run, should overall healthcare costs decrease, it should mean a decrease in taxes for the local population as well as lower out-of-pocket costs for patients. Barriers to the success of value-based care include environmental factors and high crime rates. It is difficult to guarantee high-quality outcomes when uncontrollable factors are involved.

Data Reporting

Data reporting is the main goal of data collection. Collected data are not useful until they have been gathered into some sort of report or cumulative representation. Reporting the data to either a clearinghouse or a vendor who will compile, scrub, and collate the data into meaningful results has significant impacts on an organization. For example, if a hospital collects readmission rates and reports the data to a clearinghouse who compare the rates against similar local hospitals, they may find that their rates are higher than the benchmark and will develop an action plan to decrease readmission rates. Data reporting can increase the effectiveness of how those data can be used and help to fill in the details of underlying trends or issues.

VALIDATING CODING ACCURACY
DATA SCRUBBING

Data scrubbing is a process in which data are validated and cleaned of errors and discrepancies. This includes identifying if data are complete or if they contain blanks, typos, omissions, or other inaccurate or irrelevant parts. Data scrubbing criteria are usually preset for the data to be cleaned against the correct criteria. You would not want to scrub patient care data against patient satisfaction data, so the means in which the data are being validated is critical. Data scrubbing is most often associated with clinical coding practices or maintaining accuracy in databases. When data scrubbing occurs and issues are identified, it offers time to reconcile or correct the anomalies, thus improving the quality of the data and the accuracy of the reporting outcomes.

CODING ACCURACY

Coding accuracy directly impacts billing and reimbursement. When coding practices are accurate and timely, the organization can bill and be reimbursed in a timely fashion. Multiple days may be spent attempting to code a stay because of incomplete and illegible documentation in addition to a lack of understanding of the medical terminology. This has a direct and significant impact on the timeliness of reimbursement.

However, there are several ways to increase and maintain coding accuracy efforts, for example, by ensuring that coders receive the appropriate level of training by establishing policies and investing in their continuing education. Codes are updated or reviewed frequently, so staff should receive ongoing education to stay informed. It is equally important to ensure that direct care staff are trained to document thoroughly according to state and federal guidelines. Scrubbing data and conducting regular quality audits will also help to identify coding errors early and offer time for correction before billing takes place.

IMPROPER CODING

Improper coding because of fundamental knowledge gaps or misunderstandings of coding principles and guidelines could have more than just monetary impacts. For instance, the absence of a medical coding modifier could result in an unnecessary radiology exam causing the patient out-of-pocket expenses or increasing insurance payer's costs, but it could also result in patient care errors at another treatment facility. On a larger scale, improper coding, if not quickly identified and corrected, could result in fines; accusations of fraud; being removed from private, state, or federal reimbursement programs; or removal of grants and other funding sources. It is critical to have successful auditing and monitoring programs to ensure proper and accurate coding practices.

PRIMARY DIAGNOSIS

The primary diagnosis is the established condition that, after study, was the precipitant or the primary cause for the patient's admission to the hospital. According to AHIMA and official coding guidelines, the primary diagnosis is listed first and is considered the principal diagnosis. Suppose a patient presented to the ER with the following symptoms: headaches, elevated temperature, cough, and chest pain. After the ER physician conducted a chest x-ray, lab work, and an ECG, he was able to rule out a heart attack and diagnosed the patient with congestive heart failure, resulting in an admission to the hospital. Although she presented to the ER because of her symptoms, the primary diagnosis code would be a congestive heart failure-related code because that is the condition that was identified after all of the tests and studies. Often, reimbursement programs are derived from an understanding of the analysis of an organization's principal diagnoses.

Health Plan Clinical Documentation Requirements

Referral

A referral is a request for collaborative review, consultation, studies, or some other kind of action. Referrals are often required by private or federal payers to ensure that the additional studies, tests, or consultations are medically necessary. Modern payers encourage patients to be fully involved in their care, and if patients have an ailment needing attention, they are free to seek services at the provider of their choice. For example, an individual with significant joint pain is free to bypass his or her primary care provider and seek treatment directly from an orthopedist. Some referrals are of a non-direct care method, including tobacco or substance-abuse treatment and mental health or other psychological or behavioral health consultations.

Clinical and Technical Denial

A technical denial is a denial of payment by a payer due to the healthcare provider's inability or lack of response to substantiate the services they are seeking payment for. These are easily overturned by simply proving that the services were rendered. Improving documentation quality or release of information workflows will assist with decreasing or eliminating technical denials.

A clinical denial is a denial of payment based on the lack of documentation or proof for needed services, an inability to meet medical necessity for LOS, or level-of-care efforts were exhausted. For example, Mary was approved for a 4-day psychiatric stay. Her full LOS was 7 days. The payer may deny payment for the last 3 days of her stay. Because most clinical denials can be appealed, it is essential to have staff who are knowledgeable in how to handle denials when they are received by the facility.

Payment Integrity Practices

The goal of payment integrity practices is to ensure that the payments received by payers are for the actual patients and actual services rendered. Assurances that billing practices are accurate and within the contractual or program guidelines outlined in specific payment structures is also crucial to managing payment integrity. Suppose that Sally, while processing patient bills from last month, fails to identify that two bills are duplicated and both are sent to the payer for reimbursement. A month later, while reconciling payments, she ignores the fact that the payer paid both bills and considers this a win for the hospital. This could leave the hospital open to unnecessary risk. Improving payment integrity practices and ensuring that they are honored will reduce waste, the risk of fraud, and monetary takebacks as well as fundamentally improve the quality of billing and payment activities.

E&M Coding Practices

Evaluation and management (E&M) coding is a coding type that is primary used in outpatient provider practices for billing patient encounters. E&M codes are accepted for reimbursement by private, state, and federal payers and are usually at a contracted rate. E&M coding guidelines are primarily based on four elements: the history of the present illness, a problem-focused or expanded history, the physical examination and findings, and the plan for care. Some E&M codes are based solely on time; for example, a provider spent 30 minutes with a patient for individual therapy — that individual therapy would result in a code of 90832, whereas a code for family therapy may be 90846. E&M coding guidelines are critical when it comes to who is performing the service (e.g., a physician, therapist, or nurse practitioner) as well as the setting or service location (e.g., office, home, hospital, or telehealth).

Clinical Documentation Improvement (CDI)
Physician Query

A physician query is a quality coding activity that formally asks clarifying questions to the attending physician to ensure the accuracy of coding practices. There are official query guidelines that specify that the question to the provider must not be leading or encouraging the provider toward one code or another. Doing so could be considered fraudulent because one coding structure could result in a higher reimbursement than another. A physician query should be professional, concise, and clear with consistent labeling or descriptions of the coding guidelines that the coder is investigating; the question part of the query should be last. The following is an example of a multiple-choice query:

Dr. Wells, in your 7/14 progress note you documented anemia and ordered the patient a blood transfusion. The 7/12 lab results also indicate a decrease in hematocrit that did not increase in the 7/15 and 7/20 labs. Please document which of the following type(s) of anemia you were treating this patient for:

- Sickle cell anemia
- Hemolytic anemia
- Aplastic anemia
- Another type of anemia

In response to the query example, the physician will not only review his documentation and lab work, but she may also review the supporting documents before writing a short response answering the question. Although there are no requirements related to how a physician should respond to coding questions, responses should be formalized and should offer enough clarity for coding accuracy.

Interdisciplinary Education

Interdisciplinary education entails opportunities from more than just one healthcare authority in order to obtain many perspectives. In other words, when a documentation deficiency is trending up and needs correction, it is beneficial to not only educate the prescribers but also the surgeons, nurses, therapists, unit secretaries, and members of leadership to ensure that all parties are privy to the edit and can monitor compliance while also gaining an understanding as to why the error could be occurring under the circumstances. HIM leadership will often identify those training needs and opportunities and ensure that all disciplines that need to be are educated.

Ethical Perspective to CDI

Ethics is a set of guiding principles that inform and encourage right actions. For instance, suppose Mary is performing a clinical documentation improvement (CDI) analysis on a medical record and allows one provider to document a suicide risk assessment outside the scope of the facility expectations resulting in poor patient care and poor patient outcomes. In this example, the analyst understands the importance of the assessment and understands the facility's expectations, yet she chooses to ignore documentation improvement opportunities. This would be a violation of ethics. Medical record documentation is concrete when it comes to a quantitative review; however, when it comes to a qualitative analysis, the review is more subjective, meaning that the way in which the analyst interprets the quality of the documentation has an ethical component.

Relation Between CDI and Revenue Cycle

A successful revenue cycle begins with successful coding and billing practices; neither can be successful without CDI. Because CDI strives to always have consistent, accurate, reliable, and thorough documentation to support coding and billing workflows, the relationship between the two is undeniable. Consider the following scenario: Mary is consistently only able to code records that fall into one specific diagnosis-related group, which results in a low reimbursement. She has created CDI workshops to assist physicians with clearer and more concise documentation practices. By improving the documentation and reducing the number of physician queries, she hopes to increase the coding quality and improve diagnosis-related-group assignments to, in turn, result in higher reimbursements. It is crucial for providers and members of leadership to listen to and support CDI recommendations and feedback because it is so closely tied to revenue cycle activities.

Claims Management Process
Reimbursement and Reimbursement Outliers

Reimbursement is monies paid from a payer to an organization for services rendered. Reimbursement rates are usually contractual or are driven by federal regulation and rules or other state or federal incentive programs. The reimbursement rates could vary depending on the services, tests, or procedures provided; supplies used; or even diagnoses or co-occurring conditions. The reimbursement rate for Current Procedural Terminology (CPT) codes, procedural codes used to describe the services provided, may vary from one payer to another but should remain the same within that payer's contract.

Whenever an **outlier**, or an inconsistent finding, is identified, it is important to review its cause. This could be a reimbursement that is too low or too high compared to other expected payments for the same rendered service. A simple cause for this scenario could be a clerical error or a **single-case agreement**, which is where the payer has agreed to a different payment structure that is outside the typical patient contract as part of a singular case scenario.

Payer

A payer is defined as a commercial insurance company or other type of private or federal insurance plan that pays for services rendered for their client, the patient. Depending on the facility's specialty and the services provided, the overall costs for those services are developed and monitored by federal agencies such as CMS or by contract agreements. When reviewing contracts with your highest payer, you will want to understand the case mix for whom the payer covers. For instance, when preparing for this year's budget, ABC Facility reviews the reimbursements from last year in which they received monies for 150 Medicare patients, 250 Medicaid patients, 550 patients who had either private or commercial insurance, 120 patients with self-pay, and 3 patients with single-case agreements as a result of being out of network. Associating reimbursements to each payer type will assist an organization with budget planning and identifying where contract renegotiations are needed.

Case Mix

A case mix is a description of a patient population using specific criteria such as age, gender, diagnosis, insurance, risk factors, etc. When either preparing for contract renewals or analyzing relative weights dictated by the federal register, it is important to know certain details about the patients within certain groupings. Identifying the case mix and the corresponding financial information will assist the strategic planning and budgeting of an organization. Consider the following potential scenarios at a facility:

- Cardiac patients result in a higher reimbursement than obstetrics patients, but the facility sees 20% more obstetrics patients than cardiac patients.
- Patients between the ages of 45 and 65 have a higher utilization of services rate than patients between the ages of 25 and 44.

Understanding case mix information like this will help identify whether a facility should increase offered services, eliminate a service or program, or restructure aspects of the business in order to best meet the needs of the patient population.

COLLECTIONS PROCESS

Collections is a patient accounts activity that transitions accounts that have not been paid into a more stringent workflow to attempt to collect money owed to the facility. The collection department takes rigorous steps and stronger attempts to collect past-due amounts. Those attempts may be an increase in mailings to the patient, an increase in phone calls to contact the patient, an attempt to work out a payment plan or other repayment strategies, negotiations, or settlements. Some organizations outsource their collections efforts so on-site staff can focus on current billing and account activities. Although collections has a negative connotation, facilities can work with the patient to ensure that the retrieval of late money is compassionate and understanding, while also being strategic and methodical.

DIAGNOSIS AND PROCEDURE CODE GROUPINGS

CODING SYSTEMS

Just like there are various payer types, reimbursement strategies, and contractual agreements, there are also several different coding systems. The various coding systems are evidence-based, widely used and recognized systems in the reimbursement process for large healthcare entities, as well as small practices. Depending on the entity, the specialties or services provided will depend on the coding system used. Although there are other coding systems, the following are the most prevalent systems and their primary uses:

1. **E&M codes:** derived from CPT coding structures and are primarily used to code for office visits, examinations, and tests in small practice settings.
2. **ICD-10-CM and ICD-10-PCS codes:** released by the NCHS, ICD codes are used for inpatient diagnostic and procedure coding.
3. **CPT/HCPCS codes:** released by the AMA, CPT coding is used for medical, surgical, and diagnostic services in the outpatient setting. The Healthcare Common Procedure Coding System (HCPCS) is an adoption of the CPT coding used by CMS.
4. **DSM-5:** released by the AMA are codes primarily used for psychiatric and behavior health settings.

CODING MODIFIERS

A coding modifier is a two-digit code added onto the end of CPT or HCPCS codes to indicate that a procedure or service has been altered by a specific circumstance that is slightly different than the primary code. For example, a mental health evaluation is 90791. Simply adding a -GT or -95 modifier will indicate to the payer that the mental health evaluation was conducted over a telehealth model rather than in person. Another example would be modifier 23, which can only be used with specific anesthesia codes to indicate that general anesthesia needed to be used rather than the typical local or regional block-type anesthesia. Because modifiers add related or specified conditions to the original code, it is critical to have coders understand how and when to use them. Omitting a modifier when one was required can result in a denial of claims or a loss of dollars to the organization. Coding clinics are often available to discuss the use, importance, and function of coding modifiers.

CODING CLINIC

Coding clinics are continuing education opportunities presented by local, state, or national HIM associations. Coding is a unique and specialized field in which codes are constantly being updated, removed, or added based on changes within the healthcare industry. With the ongoing discovery of new injuries, illnesses, and procedures, it is critical for healthcare entities to support the continuing education of their coders financially and otherwise.

At a typical coding clinic, presenters will share deidentified test cases to walk coders through the proper coding principles and practices of that chart. The cases are usually complex, resulting in several diagnosis and procedure codes. Ensuring that a facility's coders are up to date on code revisions and knowledgeable in their areas of expertise will result in successful and quality coding practices.

BUNDLING

While following fundamental coding guidelines, private, local, state, and federal payers will outline when it is or is not appropriate to bundle services. **Bundling** is a way to reduce the number of bills that are being sent out for a particular visit. Primarily, bundling is permitted under CPT or HCPCS coding practices. It involves billing for smaller procedures or services when they are needed or required as part of the later procedure or service. For example, a magnetic resonance imaging (MRI) scan was bundled with the larger procedure code of a knee replacement because the MRI was required and medically necessary to perform a successful surgery. Unbundling would consist of billing for the MRI and the knee replacement surgery separately. It is critical to follow the coding and payer guidelines for bundling circumstances. Not doing so could be considered upcoding and would be fraudulent.

REVENUE INTEGRITY ACTIVITIES

REVENUE INTEGRITY

Revenue integrity requires consistency to ensure ethical, accurate, and well-maintained coding, billing, and reimbursement practices. Revenue integrity is achieved through repetitive actions that are in line with personal and professional values, methods, measurements, and expected outcomes. Consider the following situation: Sal has achieved high productivity each month due to the low number of billing and reimbursement errors that he finds in the revenue cycle process. However, Sal knows that the documentation and coding practices that he is using to bill and get reimbursed are not the greatest. Revenue integrity would consist of Sal pointing out to leadership that improvements could be made to ensure that the quality of the revenue cycle is sustainable. There must be integrity checks at each point in the revenue cycle to ensure that the full process is sustaining high-quality, nonfraudulent outcomes.

HEALTHCARE REVENUE CYCLE

A revenue cycle in health care is a set of sequential steps taken to bill for patient services and then receive payment for those services. The typical steps of a revenue cycle start at the patient encounter. The patient is referred to and receives a service at a facility. The patient's insurance or payment source is verified, and, depending on the payer, authorization for those services is acquired. A physician order or referral to perform the service may be required. Once services are rendered and are coded appropriately, the bill is prepared and sent to the payer. At this point, the payer can deny the claim under a technical or clinical denial or pay the claim. Many patient accounts will be at different parts of the revenue cycle process, so it is critical to have knowledgeable and well-trained staff or a revenue cycle subcommittee to ensure that accounts are moving seamlessly through the process.

CHARGEMASTER

A chargemaster is a database monitored and maintained by the HIM, IT, and accounting departments. It is a centralized and standardized location for all billable services, medications, and supplies, and it is used to streamline and prepare reimbursement claims. The database typically outlines the charge code, CPT/HCPCS code associated with the service, item or service description, code in which the dollars are associated, and then a ledger code or which department will receive the funds. Below is a simplified sample of a chargemaster database.

Charge Code	Description	CPT Code	Revenue Code	G/L Key	Effective Date
123456	DEXA scan	77080	152	12	1/1/2020

In this example, the charge code is simply an identification number for a dual-energy x-ray absorptiometry (DEXA) scan and the associated CPT code. A revenue code is a three-digit code assigned by Medicare and is associated with reimbursement. General ledger (G/L) is an accounting term, and 12 may indicate the radiology department. The effective date is when that charge code became permissible to bill under.

MONITORING CONSIDERATIONS TO ENSURE SUCCESSFUL REVENUE CYCLE

The revenue cycle has many processes that are unique and are often dependent on the step prior to or after them. When monitoring the success or to identify potential problems in the revenue cycle, it is important to collect and trend data on the average number of days to drop a bill and on the average number of days that an account is in accounts receivable. This is essentially a measure of what the entity has billed but not received payment for.

Another critical consideration is monitoring the type and percentage of denials and then plotting them against the number of cases or admissions. When claims are going through the denial process, the entity has not been paid. When there are potential coding errors, a bill hold is initiated and claims cannot be sent to the payer. Considering all of these factors will ensure a successful revenue cycle.

Additionally, it may be beneficial to outsource the revenue cycle process to a specialty firm. To make that decision, it is critical to understand the costs associated with running the revenue cycle using in-house staff because it may or may not be cheaper to outsource the activity.

FRAUD PREVENTION
HEALTHCARE FRAUD

Healthcare fraud goes beyond inappropriate coding and billing practices: it is illegal. In health care, fraud is typically identified through routine audits or anonymous staff who abide by an ethical obligation to shed light on illegal practices. Some examples of healthcare fraud could include medical identify theft, upcoding, unbundling services, kickbacks (money earned for referrals), billing for services that were not rendered, or more services than were rendered. Insufficient monitoring practices on waste or abuse in the accounting and billing realms could be considered fraudulent because monitoring activities would have proactively identified the fraud.

FRAUD IN HIM

HIM departments must constantly monitor for fraud. Most HIM department staff have access to enormous amounts of information due to the nature of their work. Identity theft could become a problem when staff are working with patient social security numbers, off-site storage, and historical files. Staff working with patient accounts will gain access to payment sources such as credit card numbers. Chart analysts must be monitored to ensure that they are not writing in, correcting, or making other markings in the medical record, which could result in upcoding. Coders must be monitored to ensure that their physician queries are not leading questions and are written appropriately. Clear and concise policy, procedures, and training must be written such that it is understood by all staff that fraudulent activities will not be tolerated and will be grounds for termination.

UPCODING

Upcoding is an illegal practice in assigning a diagnosis that results in a higher reimbursement than what was medically necessary or properly documented. For instance, suppose an annual physical visit is coded as being more complex than what the documentation presents and what occurred. At times, a payer may become aware of upcoding when a patient is being asked to pay a deductible for a 5-minute appointment but the claim that was submitted to the payer was for a 30-minute appointment. Payers will often conduct periodic audits to ensure that coding practices match the documentation and medical necessity principles in the record. Upcoding is considered fraudulent, and it is critical to ensure that coding practices are audited for compliance.

EMR DOCUMENTATION AND PREVENTING FRAUD

The EMR can help prevent fraudulent activities because of its metadata and functionality to document each entry. The activity of making a correction in an EMR is tracked far more accurately than it is in a paper record. One cannot simply tear out and redocument in the EMR because versioning is tracked. Tables and interfaces in the EMR will ensure that documentation being added to the patient record is sufficient to support billing practices. Access auditing monitors staff involvement in and access to medical records. Therefore, it is easier to identify when a staff member is accessing a record inappropriately. EMRs also have in-program scrubbing and validation rules to help support accurate documentation, coding, and billing practices.

Management and Leadership

STRATEGIES TO SUPPORT ORGANIZATIONAL INITIATIVES
PDCA Cycle

The **PDCA cycle** is a repetitive cycle that supports continued quality improvement goals and initiatives. Regardless of the improvement focus, the PDCA cycle can be used to solve problems or to review current processes.

P = Plan: Identify the scope of the project, outline the goal or expectation of the project, and create a committee.

D = Do: Execute your plan or project. Design, build, and implement the forms or tools needed for success.

C = Check: Once implemented, check, monitor, and audit for quality or hindrances.

A = Act: Create an action plan with the findings from the check section. Act on that action plan. Retrain staff, redesign forms, and adjust the process as needed.

At times, an "**O**" **for observation** is placed in the PDCA cycle model if it has become evident that change cannot occur without current observations of the problem or significant observations during the check step. No quality improvement PDCA cycle will be perfectly successful the first time around; that is why the cycle repeats.

Supporting Organizational Initiatives at the Department Level

Not all staff are privy to all larger organizational initiatives. High-level organizational initiatives are at times too complex and comprehensive for staff. Some initiatives are more than improving customer service scores through front desk friendliness. For example, although an HIM clerk may not know that the hospital where they work is seeking Joint Commission accreditation, their involvement is vital in achieving that goal by successfully performing their job duties. When trying to achieve a larger organizational initiative at the department level, it is critical for department leaders to hold meetings with staff to set clear, achievable goals and expectations and to communicate how achieving the department's goals will help achieve the larger objective. Organizational initiatives are not achieved quickly; therefore, holding staff accountable for their part in the department's success will play a large role in the overall success of the initiative.

Staff Involvement

Involving staff in the discussion, planning, or implementation of organizational initiatives is critical to ensure the success of those initiatives. Leaders can solidify staff involvement through regular staff meetings to maintain transparency, offer town halls with leadership to help explain the initiative and elicit staff input, incentivize their involvement, and encourage peer support or recognition. Because staff are the ones executing the initiatives in their daily work, it is critical to ensure their support and involvement. Suppose that a hospital changes their telephone etiquette policy in hopes that it will increase customer satisfaction scores. They do not explain this or elicit staff involvement, so front-line staff have no context or interest in supporting the policy change. Organizational initiatives will become burdensome and fail if staff do not believe in the goal, or if they do not have a clear understanding of the reason for an action or requirement. One way to aid in this process is to develop staff ambassadors who become the trailblazers for change and help to ensure the overall success of strategies and facility initiatives.

Department Meetings to Support Organizational Initiatives

At times, an organization or their initiatives are too large, or they are too widespread to elicit a functional and productive subcommittee. For example, ABC Hospital has 12 satellite facilities impeding a quick rollout of a strategic initiative. Wishing to maintain staff involvement, leadership regularly schedules staff or department meetings to offer time to hear staff ideas, concerns, questions, and clarifications. The department heads then share the staff feedback to the senior leaders trying to implement the initiative. Ideally, once the senior leaders have initiated change or made some other kind of progress toward their goal, a deadline can be set for all department heads to roll that information down to their staff. This process can repeat until the initiative is fully implemented. Aside from organizational initiatives, department meetings are a great way to continue the growth of a professional relationship and trust between leaders and their staff.

Contract Management
Vendor Quality Reviews

A **vendor** is a person or business that performs a service for or sells something to the organization. A vendor may or may not also be a business associate depending on the service provided, and may or may not have access to and use of PHI. Regardless of the vendor type, it is important to perform periodic quality audits to be sure that the vendor is continuously providing quality services and upholding other contractual terms. Consider a situation revealed by a quality audit: a technician working for a laboratory vendor has not been applying the two patient identifiers before drawing blood and reportedly has not greeted patients professionally. The laboratory tech is performing a service under contract terms that include professionalism and should be held to the same standards as on-site staff and is therefore in breach of that contract. The behaviors may warrant retraining or disciplinary action. Performing quality reviews of contracted workflows or services will help evaluate whether the contract should be renewed or renegotiated. Any noncompliance, especially when the vendor is also a business associate under HIPAA, would result in grounds to dissolve the contract.

BAs and BA Agreements

Business associates (BAs) are other organizations, companies, or individuals that perform a service for a covered entity in which the BA uses or discloses PHI. For instance, suppose the HIM department uses an off-site storage company to outsource their release of information functions or a nursing home outsources laboratory services to the local hospital. This makes those facilities a business associate because they will be accessing, using, and disclosing patient PHI on behalf of the healthcare facility. BAs are held to the same standards as healthcare facilities under HIPAA, meaning that they must follow the rules and regulations regarding patient privacy and breach notification laws. The **BA agreement,** also required by HIPAA, will outline the covered entity's and the business associate's roles and responsibilities as they relate to patient health information.

Outsourcing

Outsourcing means delegating a task, activity, or function to another person or vendor outside the organization. That entity is then bound by contractual agreement with the organization. Under some circumstances, outsourced activities may still be performed on the grounds, but it is the outsourced vendor performing the function not the staff of the organization. Organizations typically choose to outsource to save money on the staff, supply, or operating costs associated with unique specialties or high-frequency areas such as housekeeping, maintenance, or kitchen staff.

PRIMARY FUNCTIONS OF CONTRACT MANAGEMENT

A **contract** is a legally binding agreement between two parties to engage in business: the one providing the service and the other needing and accepting the service. Contract management involves monitoring the validity of the contract terms, ensuring that the terms are being appropriately executed, and verifying that payment structures are in line with the contract. The four primary functions of contract management after identifying the need are as follows:

- Drafting and making an offer to a contractor
- Both parties accepting the terms of the contract
- Understanding the intentions of the contract
- Outlining the considerations, payment, or profit sharing for the contracted services

Contract writing and management is a valuable professional qualification because organizations will often contract with high-level accounts that impact the annual budget.

HUMAN RESOURCE MANAGEMENT ACTIVITIES
JOB DESCRIPTION

A job description is an outline of the roles, responsibilities, qualifications, and education requirements being requested or minimally required to successfully perform in a job position. Each position in an organization should be accompanied by a job description because it helps outline the expectations for that role and allows for clear and concise narrative about the job position. A job description makes it clear to job seekers what it is they are applying for and reduces the risk of the employer hiring someone who is not qualified for the position. Job descriptions are typically written by the leadership of the department and are maintained by the human resources department. Organizationally, job descriptions are tools used for performance management, recruitment, retention, and compensation comparisons.

DISCIPLINARY PROCESS

The disciplinary process is a pre-established set of actions that are taken when a staff member is continuously not meeting performance standards. A typical disciplinary process would follow these steps: verbal warning, written warning, probation, and, finally, termination. Each step in the process will have its own set of expectations and offense severity scales. For example, a verbal warning is a contact between an employer and the employee to verbally discuss an area of concern, whereas probation will hold significant consequences because it would indicate that the staff has not or will not correct their questionable practices or behaviors. Although organizations may vary on the nomenclature of the process steps, it is universal that the intention of the disciplinary process is to initiate change and correct areas of concern. Each step in the disciplinary process should be carefully carried out and documented thoroughly to maximize the effectiveness of the plan. Additionally, if a wrongful termination or discrimination lawsuit occurs, the documentation will be an essential part of the defense.

RESOLVING PERSONNEL CONFLICTS

Personnel conflicts arise when staff members experience obvious frustrations with peers that can no longer be worked out by themselves. Many things can trigger personnel conflicts, which may or may not be related to the work itself. It could simply be character flaws that another staff member can no longer tolerate. Consider the following scenario: Julie and David have been arguing throughout the day. Julie is now losing productive time because she's in the restroom collecting her emotions. As a supervising manager, the HIM director may want to sit with both employees individually to see what the triggering event was and how it could be prevented in the future. A mediation meeting between the two staff members may be needed to identify an action plan.

Resolving personnel conflicts would consist of following company policies: identifying if the triggers can be controlled or eliminated and, ideally, coming to a quick resolution so that it does not impede the other workers or their productivity.

STAFF INSUBORDINATION

Insubordination is disobedience, defiance, or continuous noncompliance against a superior. For example, a record clerk continuously refuses to organize loose reports in alphabetical order despite being asked to do so numerous times by the supervisor. Insubordination is disrespectful and commonly goes against a company's ethical and behavioral standards and expectations from staff. It can disrupt the work environment and cause conflict, detract from the quality of patient care, or impede the overall organizational or departmental functioning.

WORK DESIGN AND PROCESS IMPROVEMENT ACTIVITIES
JOB REDESIGN

Job redesign is the process by which a specific job task or set of tasks is reevaluated for effectiveness, efficiency, and expectations. For instance, if a hospital moves to an EMR, then the manual record completion job task is now obsolete. It is important for department leaders to reanalyze workflows and job tasks when tasks are outdated, obsolete, or redundant. Job redesigns may also increase staff productivity and reduce burdensome tasks, which may then allow staff to cross train in other areas of the department.

STRATEGIC THINKING

Strategic thinking incorporates critical thinking as well as considering perspectives that are new or foreign to others. When training new staff, the phrase "it has always been done this way" is a common example of nonstrategic thinking. Staff who are successful with problem solving, detail orientated, and thorough are the ones who will become highly strategic thinkers. For example, Mary, trained on the timeliness of cosigning physician orders, identifies that every record that she has analyzed is noncompliant. She begins to review the causes for the lateness and various solutions to improve the compliance rates. Strategic thinkers can also identify potential issues and brainstorm solutions before a problem actually occurs.

ENGAGING STAFF IN PI

To have a successful business and business practices, performance improvement (PI) is essential. Healthcare organizations and members of leadership may be the ones determining goals and initiatives, but it is the front-line staff who will ultimately achieve those initiatives on behalf of leadership. When engaging staff in PI projects or initiatives, it is important to have transparency. Explaining the reasons behind the initiatives will help solidify belief in the goal. This can help to engender a sense of ownership in assigned tasks, which will in turn increase the likelihood of a successful implementation of PI projects. Employees will take the additional time and effort required to do a great job if there is an association between that and feelings of achievement and accomplishment or other incentives. When staff feel motivated, there is a greater likelihood that they will work smarter, harder, and more efficiently.

CONSTRUCTIVE FEEDBACK

Constructive criticism is a supervisory action that involves a person in a supervisory role offering feedback to an employee that may be taken negatively or with offense, when it is not intended. Encouraging high staff morale can be challenging when staff do not feel supported in the workplace. Therefore, ensuring that feedback is done privately will not only improve the interaction between two parties but will also help build trust between them. Supervisors who set clear, concise, and achievable expectations from staff, with ongoing regular feedback, will get the best results from their staff.

Training and Development
Best Practices

A best practice is the most streamlined or most accepted practice in the industry to perform or complete a task. Best practices that have already been through the trial-and-error stages and consistently produce highly effective results are called **evidence-based practices**. However, the term evidence-based practice is mostly constrained to the clinical realm of health care. In the clerical and administrative aspects of health care, there are many best practices that can be applied. For example, before initiating the assembly process, it is a best practice to collect yesterday's discharges all at once during the morning hours rather than at many times throughout the day. The latter process would reduce the staff's productivity because they will need to make many trips to the units during busier staffing and visiting hours. Best practices are initiated by organizations to increase productivity, reduce operating and staff costs, and improve turnaround times.

Legal Implications of Training and Development

When human resource departments are looking at training and development plans for their staff, it is critical to understand all of the various locations in which staff members work. Not all staff will be working at a desk and with computers. Therefore, those training expectations and plans will be quite different from someone in maintenance or housekeeping, for example. Not supplying staff with proper training that matches the person's native language and learning needs, could be discriminatory and could be grounds for litigation due to inappropriate or insufficient training and development for new staff. The required training and development plan for almost all industries falls under Occupational Safety and Health Administration (OSHA) guidelines. OSHA is a regulatory agency that oversees safe working environments for all staff. Below is a sample of OSHA's training requirements:

- Knowledge of hazardous products or chemicals in work areas
- Process of tagging out a piece of faulty equipment
- Handling of blood and bloodborne pathogens
- Use of personal protective equipment for head, eyes, ears, face, and feet, etc.
- Safety incident reporting protocols
- Fall and slip prevention
- Heavy equipment usage and safety precautions

Compliance with OSHA regulations helps to ensure that all staff are safe when working.

Training and Development Plans

Training and development are important aspects of HIM departments and the overall success of the organization. Human resource departments rely on the training and development of staff to ensure their competence. Plans may consist of required annual coursework related to patient safety, environmental safety such as fire drills, cultural diversity, or mental health awareness. Job-specific training and development may consist of ongoing shadowing with a more experienced peer, coding clinics, or other continuing education to ensure job-specific competencies. Whether the hospital, department, or larger industry or specialty associations are organizing the training and development plans, there are steps that should be taken to ensure that the plans are successful, including the following:

1. Identify the training need.
2. Understand the learning curve and the needs of the trainees.
3. Write and deliver the curriculum.
4. Evaluate the effectiveness of the plan.

Ensuring the successful implementation of training and development plans will encourage employee satisfaction and longevity from staff.

EOC COMMITTEES

An environment-of-care (EOC) committee is a requirement for Joint Commission accreditation. Outlined in the Joint Commission standard EC.02.01.01 EP 1, the EOC committee's objective is to ensure that the facility's environment is conducive to safe patient care practices. An EOC committee will meet monthly to ensure that safety drills are taking place, such as fire drills or emergency response drills. They will collect data and report on unit or facility safety inspections and maintenance requests, and they will ensure that generator, HVAC, and other facility inspections are up to date and conduct risk assessments to identify vulnerabilities. Staff and patient incidents related to the facility environment may also be reported if they are environmentally related. Contract negotiations and approvals will be discussed should the contract be required for facilities or environmental care such as linens, housekeeping, or maintenance contracts.

PREPARATION OF BUDGETS
COLAS AND MARKET ADJUSTMENTS

A cost-of-living adjustment (COLA) is common during annual review of staff salaries to be sure that salaries are comparable to the cost of living in the geographic area. A **market adjustment** would be a comparison and analysis of compensation for one's roles and responsibilities against jobs with similar roles and responsibilities. Depending on the outcome of that analysis, a market adjustment to one's hourly rate or salary could be made.

Consider the following calculation of a 1% performance raise and 2% COLA, or an overall 3% increase for a staff member with an hourly rate of $15.42. Begin by converting the percentage to a decimal: 3% = 3/100 = 0.03. Then multiply this by the hourly rate: $15.42 × 0.03 = $0.46. This person is getting a $0.46 raise with the 1% for performance and the 2% COLA. Finally, add the increase to the original hourly rate: $15.42 + $0.46 = $15.88. So, the staff member's new hourly rate is $15.88.

IMPORTANCE OF TERMS OF A RAISE

It is important to be strategic about when to apply a percentage increase on top of a dollar amount increase because this will vary the final salary amount. When a dollar amount raise is being applied to a base salary, it will then change the amount at which the percentage is being applied.

Consider the following scenario: the HIM director's annual salary is $52,000. Senior leadership is giving the director a $4,000 raise and a 2% COLA. The terms of the raise are that the $4,000 be applied before the COLA is applied. Because the $4000 raise is applied first and the 2% COLA is applied after, the new salary = (base salary + raise) × COLA

$$= (\$52{,}000 + \$4{,}000) \times 1.02$$
$$= \$56{,}000 \times 1.02$$
$$= \$57{,}120$$

If the 2% COLA had been applied first and the $4000 raise applied after, then it would have resulted in a slightly lower salary:

$$\text{new salary} = (\text{base salary} \times \text{COLA}) + \text{Raise}$$
$$= (\$52{,}000 \times 1.02) + \$4{,}000$$
$$= \$53{,}040 + \$4{,}000$$
$$= \$57{,}040$$

Different Budget Lines That Would Impact an HIM Department

Although organizational budgets are created, monitored, and approved by senior leaders, departmental leadership will assist in monitoring their portions of the larger organizational budget. Typical HIM departments will have costs or budget lines associated with staff salaries, supplies, and off-site storage costs. An **operating budget** consists of those costs associated with the general and administrative expenses of the department such as salary distribution and supplies related to copy paper, toner, books, or manuals to assist with specific job duties. A **capital budget** consists of long-term investment costs, in other words, money that is budgeted for work environmental upkeep such as painting or structural projects, machinery replacement, annual maintenance fees, and large equipment purchases or repair costs. Consider the following scenario: ABC Hospital has an annual budget of $2,000,000 with the HIM department having a budget of $500,000. The HIM director is responsible for allocating and monitoring its spending. The budget may be categorized as follows:

Category	Amount
Salaries: one director and four staff	$255,000
Off-site storage and shredding	$50,000
Supplies and services	$100,000
Capital projects (new photocopier and fax machine)	$145,000

Budget Proposal

A budget proposal is an established and defined item that is being presented to a decision maker. When preparing budget proposals, it is essential to understand the current average costs for supplies and services and what was spent in the past. Consider the following scenario: historically, the HIM department spent approximately $2,500 requesting, retrieving, and storing boxes each month equaling a $30,000 annual budget. However, with the implementation of the EMR, the need for off-site storage has decreased because there are fewer paper records to be maintained. As a result, over the past 3 years, the average monthly costs were $1,300. The HIM director could prepare a proposed annual budget of $16,000 for the upcoming year given the trend of the past few years. Budget proposals are presented to organizational decision makers who understand the full scope of the strategic plan and where money needs to be allocated.

Entity Accreditation, Licensing, and Certification Processes
Focused Standards Assessment

It is good organizational practice to perform a **focused standards assessment**. In other words, an agency would routinely review their accrediting body list of standards to monitor the agency's compliance with those standards. In 2012, the Joint Commission introduced an intracycle monitoring system that continued to encourage the focused standards assessment. Facilities that are accredited by the Joint Commission should adopt and complete this self-assessment prior to an upcoming survey year. This will assist the facility and the accrediting agency in preparation for the actual survey. When a discrepancy or omission is found during a focused standard review, a subcommittee should be formed to identify the intent of the standard and how it needs to be implemented into the organization or how the organization may be exempt from that particular standard. For example, if it does not apply to the services provided at that organization.

ORGANIZATIONAL READINESS AND PREPAREDNESS PRACTICES FOR ACCREDITATION PROCESSES

Accreditation is recognition or endorsement by an agency that sets the quality-of-care standards for an entity. For hospitals, the most nationally recognized accrediting agency is the Joint Commission. Accrediting agencies each have a set of evidence-based practices and standards that a hospital must adhere to in order to be deemed a quality facility. These accrediting agencies are closely tied to federal and state agencies that assist in reimbursements and other payment initiatives. Though voluntary, without accreditation, facilities run the risk of decreased patient census and a lack of or loss of grants, donations, or federal funding. Consider the following scenario: ABC Hospital has been a Joint Commission-accredited facility for 20 years; however, they did not choose the Joint Commission as their accrediting agency this year, which resulted in a loss of $50,000 in anticipated donations. Because accreditation surveys regularly result in prestigious ratings, funding, or both, organizational preparation for an accreditation survey is critical. Rounding, staff monitoring, monthly tracers, and reviews of policy and procedures against standards are great ways to prepare for an accreditation visit.

ORGANIZATIONAL READINESS AND PREPAREDNESS PRACTICES FOR LICENSING PROCESSES

Organizational **licensing** is the legal authority and legal permissions given to an entity to perform a function or service. Organizational licensing comes from the state level and is always required to operate a healthcare facility. The state will license an entity for services that it is able to provide, approve patient capacity, and monitor the quality level at which those services and programs are being performed. State agencies will also conduct on-site or tabletop survey audits to ensure that the facility is compliant with related laws, regulations, and standards as well as the terms of the licensing. For example, if ABC Hospital is licensed to operate a facility with a 92-bed capacity, then holding a capacity larger than 92, without prior approval, would be noncompliant with state licensing and could result in repercussions. State health departments may license medical facilities, whereas state mental health agencies will license psychiatric facilities. State-level licensing audits are conducted annually, and preparation for them is conducted in the same way as accreditation preparedness, consisting of rounding, staff monitoring, and policy and procedure reviews.

ORGANIZATIONAL READINESS AND PREPAREDNESS PRACTICES FOR CERTIFICATION PROCESSES

Organizational or program **certification** is established once a predefined set of requirements and competencies has been met. This set is outlined by an authoritative or recognizable entity, often a nongovernmental agency; for example, a hospital may receive certification from the American Heart Association for readiness to treat stroke patients, or the American Board of Pediatrics may certify a hospital for readiness to treat general pediatric patients or subspecialities as they relate to pediatric patients.

On the other hand, if a cardiologist has not completed the required continuing education credits needed to maintain his physician credentials and, furthermore, patient outcome and satisfaction survey results have decreased in this particular area, this may result in a loss of certification for the hospital. In that case, the hospital will no longer be able to provide a service. Staff training, ongoing staff competencies, and ensuring that credentialed staff maintain their earned credentials are all critical when re-establishing certification for certain initiatives or services performed at a facility.

RHIA Practice Test #1

Want to take this practice test in an online interactive format?
Check out the bonus page, which includes interactive practice questions and much more: mometrix.com/bonus948/rhia

1. In ICD-10-CM, which term is used to describe "not included here"?
    a. See
    b. Excludes 1
    c. Code also
    d. Excludes 2

2. In assessing the length of time that a facility is required to maintain its records, which of the following should be the facility's first concern?
    a. The most stringent state or federal regulation
    b. The total number of records
    c. The medium in which records will be retained
    d. The cost associated with records retention

3. According to the Medicare Conditions of Participation, hospital records are required to have a _____-year retention period.
    a. 10
    b. 5
    c. 3
    d. 15

4. Which of the following is an agency that creates and maintains standards for laboratory tests and results?
    a. SNOWMED CT
    b. MEDCIN
    c. LOINC
    d. NDC

5. Which type of data is entered into registries and databases and allows users to be able to conduct trend analyses, review and establish benchmarks, and execute long-term planning?
    a. Secondary
    b. Primary
    c. Aggregate
    d. Index

6. Pathological data characterizing site, stage of neoplasm, and type of treatment would be reported in which of the following registries?
   a. Diabetes
   b. Immunization
   c. Cancer
   d. Trauma

7. The _____ organization is responsible for the creation of standards to address healthcare transactions between health partners.
   a. ANSI
   b. ASTM
   c. OASIS
   d. HL7

8. When a task requires data for detailed root cause analysis, which type of data is preferred and why?
   a. Structured data are preferred because they provide a clearer picture of the situation.
   b. Unstructured data are preferred because they allow for more granular review.
   c. Structured data are preferred because they have useful metadata to provide additional information.
   d. Unstructured data are preferred because they are easier to query and analyze.

9. A procedure involving the cutting out of solid matter is considered what root operation?
   a. Extirpation
   b. Release
   c. Detachment
   d. Destruction

10. The root operation destruction means:
    a. Freeing a body part from an abnormal physical contract by cutting or force
    b. Physical eradication of all or a portion of a body part by the direct use of energy, force, or destructive agent
    c. Taking or cutting out solid matter from body part
    d. Taking or letting out fluids and/or gases from a body part

11. The root operation release means:
    a. Cutting off without replacement
    b. Freeing a body part from an abnormal physical contract by cutting or force
    c. Cutting off with replacement
    d. Breaking solid matter into pieces

12. When destroying data in a paper format, which method is the most appropriate method?
    a. Shredding
    b. Encrypting
    c. Burning
    d. Placing information in a locked drawer away from patient access

13. If unforeseen scenarios occur such as power outages, fires, natural disasters, etc., what should facilities have in place to ensure that there are procedures to handle emergency response situations with respect to continuing operations?

    a. Disaster recovery plan
    b. Business continuity/contingency plan
    c. Training
    d. Risk and audit controls

14. Which act addressed issues with respect to the portability of health insurance after leaving employment?

    a. Affordable Care Act
    b. Omnibus Budget Reconciliation Act
    c. Health Insurance Portability and Accountability Act
    d. Health Information Technology for Economic and Clinical Health (HITECH) Act

15. All of the following are data security functions of data governance EXCEPT:

    a. Identifying and resolving quality issues
    b. Establishing a risk-management program
    c. Implementing security awareness for employees
    d. Facility data security planning

16. The process of defining levels of data quality by establishing parameters to ensure that the data meet business needs is:

    a. Data security management
    b. Terminology and classification management
    c. Content management
    d. Data quality management

17. Qualitative analysis performed after a patient has been discharged and reviewed retrospectively is:

    a. Open-record review
    b. Closed-record review
    c. Discharged-patient review
    d. Retro-quality review

18. What is the standards development organization that develops messaging, data content, and document standards to improve the exchange of clinical information?

    a. IEEE
    b. HL7
    c. ADA
    d. ISO

19. Within entity relationship modeling, what is the process by which entity relationship diagrams are converted into tables?

    a. Schema mapping
    b. Cardinality
    c. Attributes
    d. Normalization

20. A discrepancy is found in which a patient's birthdate is listed as 07/12/2008 on one record and as 09/12/2008 on another record. Which characteristic of data quality does this discrepancy represent?

   a. Precision
   b. Granularity
   c. Consistency
   d. Timeliness

21. A pediatrician would like to report hydrocephalus in a newborn. To which registry would reporting this information be most relevant?

   a. Diabetes
   b. Immunization
   c. Birth defect
   d. Trauma

22. Creating and revising information within a patient's progress note is whose responsibility?

   a. Administrator
   b. Health information management (HIM) professional
   c. Registration staff
   d. Provider

23. What is the legal document that designates another person to act on behalf of the patient in the event that the patient becomes disabled and/or incapacitated?

   a. Living will
   b. Durable power of attorney
   c. Informed consent
   d. Health Insurance Portability and Accountability Act of 1996 (HIPAA) form

24. Where are guidelines for the retention and destruction of healthcare information found?

   a. Accreditation standards
   b. HIPAA
   c. HITECH Act
   d. Articles of participation

25. The focus of a certified coder is geared toward which of the following?

   a. Ensure maximum reimbursement
   b. Avoid coding claim edits
   c. Avoid write-offs due to claim rejections
   d. Ensure that each claim is coded with accuracy

26. Data found in patient/disease registries are considered to be which of the following?

   a. Financial data
   b. Clinical data
   c. Demographic data
   d. Accreditation data

27. _____ typically occurs when there is a transfer of data between systems. This is most often seen when companies are implementing new systems.
    a. Data dictionary analysis
    b. Data mining
    c. Data migration
    d. Data analysis

28. Procedures that include the altering of a route of passage of contents of a tubular body part is which of the following root operations?
    a. Dilation
    b. Fragmentation
    c. Occlusion
    d. Bypass

29. What is the overall goal of documenting and maintaining medical records?
    a. To ensure that clean claims are sent in order to provide maximum reimbursement
    b. To provide data to avoid malpractice issues
    c. To aid in the continuity of care
    d. To adhere to guidelines set forth by the American Health Information Management Association (AHIMA)

30. Records arranged in strict chronological order are considered to be which of the following?
    a. Source-oriented health records
    b. Problem-oriented medical records
    c. Integrated health records
    d. Ascending health records

31. Which of the following is NOT considered clinical data?
    a. Medical history
    b. Physical exam
    c. Diagnostic orders
    d. A patient's hospital unique identifier

32. Who is responsible for setting the strategic direction of the hospital?
    a. Chief executive officer
    b. Board of directors
    c. Chief nursing officer
    d. Chief information officer

33. Which law is considered "unwritten" law originating from previous court decisions?
    a. Common law
    b. Constitutional law
    c. Administrative law
    d. Statutory law

34. Who does ownership of health records ultimately belong to?
   a. The patient
   b. U.S. Department of Health and Human Services (HHS)
   c. Office for Civil Rights (OCR)
   d. The organization that created and maintained the physical record

35. Managing the input of data is defined as:
   a. Data governance
   b. Information governance
   c. Data quality management
   d. Data enterprise management

36. Managing the output of data is defined as:
   a. Data governance
   b. Information governance
   c. Data quality management
   d. Data enterprise management

37. If more than _____ individuals have been affected by a breach, the media as well as the HHS must be notified.
   a. 500
   b. 100
   c. 50
   d. 350

38. The HIPAA Security Rule contains two standards: _____ and _____. One standard is mandated, and organizations must adhere to the standard as written under the HIPAA Security Rule; the other standard provides flexibility to covered entities.
   a. required, nonrequired
   b. required, addressable
   c. mandatory, tentative
   d. mandatory, addressable

39. Which type of safeguard includes encryption, decryption, and automatic logoff?
   a. Physical
   b. Technical
   c. Administrative
   d. Privacy

40. In instances in which federal and state laws conflict, what law takes precedence?
   a. The most stringent of the laws is what prevails.
   b. Federal law always prevails over state law.
   c. State law always prevails over federal law.
   d. Facilities are allowed to choose which law prevails as long as they are consistently applying the law.

41. All of the following are identifiers under the HIPAA Privacy Rule EXCEPT:
   a. Social security numbers
   b. Gender
   c. Admission date
   d. Birth date

42. Which federal law provides standards related to physician peer review and also provides legal immunity to other physicians who participate in peer review activity?
   a. HIPAA
   b. The HITECH Act
   c. The Healthcare Quality Improvement Act
   d. The National Practitioner Data Bank

43. Dominique is a director exploring the causes and effects associated with opening up a new clinic for psychiatric services. Which visual tool will best represent Dominique's need?
   a. Pareto chart
   b. Fishbone diagram
   c. Flowchart
   d. Bar graph

44. Cassidy is participating in a research study. She is asked to sign an informed consent form in order to go through with the treatment in the study. Cassidy has agreed to sign the form. Per HIPAA requirements, which of the following is correct?
   a. The investigator has completed his or her due diligence in receiving the informed consent document from Cassidy.
   b. The investigator has received the informed consent form; however, this alone does not constitute an adequate consent process.
   c. The investigator has asked Cassidy to sign the form in error because research study participants are not required to sign the form.
   d. The investigator should have retrieved this form from Cassidy as well as the study sponsor to fully abide by HIPAA guidelines.

45. Dr. Zane makes an agreement to refer patients to Dr. McCarthy in return for a specified compensation amount per patient. Although Dr. Zane believes this is illegal, Dr. McCarthy assures him that this is not illegal in that the referrals are only done for the continuity of care and in the patients' best interests. Is there a law prohibiting the actions mentioned above, and, if so, what is it called?
   a. Yes, the agreement between the two physicians is considered illegal by violating the Anti-referral Act of 1997.
   b. No, the agreement is not illegal due to the fact that the referral is made with continuity of care in mind.
   c. Yes, the agreement between the two physicians is considered illegal by violating the Stark Law.
   d. No, the agreement is not illegal due to permissions set forth by the Sherman Anti-Trust Act, which allows for compensation of referrals when it is in the best interest of the patient.

46. Daisy has requested a copy of her PHI from the Scott Chiropractic Center. It has been 7 years since she has been seen at this practice. She is told that although maintained, she will not be able to receive her records due to the fact that the records are more than 5 years old. By law, what are the parameters around patients' ability to receive their records?

   a. Access is granted up to 5 years from the last documented activity on the patient's account.
   b. As long as the records are being maintained by the facility, patients should have rights to access.
   c. Records are available for patient access for 24 months from the last date of service.
   d. Patients must be able to access their records for an indefinite period of time.

47. A patient has been deemed mentally incompetent, and her niece has requested her medical records on her behalf. The patient's niece has not been identified as the legal guardian for the patient nor has she provided any legal documentation in support of her efforts. A fully compliant facility will handle this scenario in which of the following ways?

   a. Provide records to the niece depending on urgency of request.
   b. Inform the niece that they are unable to provide medical records for any circumstance unless authorization of the release is obtained by the patient regardless of competency.
   c. Inform the niece that a one-time release of medical records will be granted due to the incompetency status of her relative.
   d. Inform the niece that they will not be releasing medical records to her at this time, and advise her to seek legal means if she is now the guardian of her aunt.

48. What is considered to be the legal age of majority?

   a. 18 and over — this is federally mandated and is standard across states.
   b. 18 and over — however, this may vary from state to state.
   c. 21 and over — this is federally mandated and is consistent across states.
   d. 16 and over — this is federally mandated and is consistent across states.

49. A 13-year-old child has been seen by a neurology practice in the month of December. The child's parents are divorced, and the mother has requested that the father not have access to the child's records at any time. Is the facility able to honor her request?

   a. No, with no legal documentation stating that the biological father cannot have access or involvement in medical decision making for the child, the mother has no rights to eliminate the father from being able to request medical documentation on the child.
   b. Yes, parents have the right to restrict other parents from release of medical records on children if the parent requesting the restriction has the child living in their care for more than half the year.
   c. Yes, in divorce situations, the mother is given the decision-making privileges in respect to medical release for the children.
   d. Yes, as long as her request is in writing and notarized.

50. At Midtown Heart Clinic, a patient complained that during his first visit with the facility he was not made aware of the facility's notice of privacy practice (NPP), although he signed the NPP form. He stated that because the NPP was not located on display within the waiting area that he would escalate his complaint with governing bodies as a HIPAA violation. Which of the following is true regarding NPPs?

    a. All NPPs must be located in common areas within the facility as well as provided in paper format when coming to the practice as a new patient.
    b. NPPs must be signed by each patient upon first visiting the practice and must be mailed regularly to patients for awareness.
    c. NPPs must be reasonably placed in prominent areas of the facilities and must be signed on new-patient visits, as well as sent to established patients when changes are made to the document.
    d. NPPs are only required to be distributed on an annual basis regardless of patient status or changes to the document.

51. The Walter MacDonald Urology Clinic often refers its patients to Cedar Hospital for further evaluation in the transferring of care. Both facilities are governed by HIPAA regulations and are considered to be which of the following?

    a. Managed-care entities
    b. Regulated parties
    c. Covered entities
    d. Third-party covered agents

52. Macom Physician Practice does not require its employees to lock file cabinets that contain patient PHI. This could potentially be an issue for the practice and cause issues with violating HIPAA regulations. This scenario is an example of which of the following?

    a. Vulnerability
    b. Threat
    c. Breach
    d. Incident

53. Why is the role of the database administrator significant in respect to user access?

    a. There is no significance because a database administrator would not be involved with user access. This would be the data analyst.
    b. Database administrators grant user access using role-based methodology within a facility to protect unauthorized users from accessing information that is not required by their roles.
    c. The database administrator works under the director of HIM, and he or she executes decisions on user access made by the director to determine which users have access to certain parts of the system.
    d. There is no significance because the database administrator would not be involved with user access. Access is granted by the director of HIM per manager request.

54. How is the Medicare Conditions of Participation: Confidentiality of patient records, related to the HIPAA Privacy Rule?

a. Medicare Conditions of Participation: Confidentiality of patient records, is found within the HIPAA Privacy Rule.
b. The HIPAA Privacy Rule was implemented as a result of the Medicare Conditions of Participation.
c. There is no relation between the two: Both regulations relate to two mutually exclusive topics within HIM.
d. Medicare Conditions of Participation: Confidentiality of patient records and the HIPAA Privacy Rule requirements are consistent in meaning, defining actions, and intent.

55. In review of the disclosure and redisclosure of confidential health information, an HIM employee states that both should be handled in the same manner according to regulatory guidelines. Do you agree or disagree with the employee? How would you outline your response to the employee?

a. Agree. Disclosures and redisclosures involve the same elements and are governed according to the same regulatory guidelines.
b. Agree. Although disclosure and redisclosure involve different elements, they are governed by the same regulatory guidelines.
c. Disagree. Disclosures and redisclosures consist of different elements; therefore, they are governed by different regulatory guidelines.
d. Disagree. Disclosures and redisclosures consist of the same elements; however, they are governed by different regulatory guidelines.

56. What is the correlation between retention rates of records and the statute of limitations?

a. The terms retention rate and statute of limitations, in respect to records, are synonymous in most states.
b. Retention rates are established by each state; however, if a state does not have a specific retention rate, the state's statute of limitation may be used as law.
c. The statute of limitations overrides established retention rates in a court of law and must be followed if mandated by a state.
d. States must abide by the longer time frame between the established retention rate and defined law around the statute of limitations.

57. Per the HIPAA Security Rule, there are three safeguards: administrative, physical, and technical. What information would an HIM employee need to make a decision about whether or not a medical center had sufficient physical safeguards?

a. Review of policies and procedures to address authorized and unauthorized facility access to electronic information systems and facilities where the information is being stored
b. Review of policies and procedures to protect ePHI and access control
c. Review of policies and procedures related to the privacy and confidentiality of information
d. Review of policies outlining the center's approach to risk management and risk analysis

58. An audit is performed to review Staples Medical Center's process for the destruction of records. The employees inform the auditor that they currently have issues finding effective ways of documenting the destruction of records. They also explain that when they do document, they keep their documentation on file for 7 years. This mirrors their retention policy. From the viewpoint of the auditor, what recommendations would you give to the medical center?
   a. To keep destruction-of-records documentation within an Excel file that is saved on site as well as backed up to an offsite database. The destruction-of-records documentation filing for 7 years is acceptable because it mirrors the center's retention policy.
   b. To keep destruction-of-records documentation within an Excel file that is saved on site as well as backed up to an offsite database, but to also recommend that per the guidelines, destruction-of-records documentation should be kept permanently.
   c. To keep destruction-of-records documentation in the form of destruction certificates and to keep the documentation permanently.
   d. To keep destruction-of-records documentation in the form of destruction certificates. The destruction-of-records documentation filing for 7 years is acceptable because it mirrors the center's retention policy.

59. Charlotte in the HIM Department would like to speak to Frank, the revenue manager, about a trend found within the documentation coming out of the Cardiology Department. Charlotte sent patient examples to Frank's work email with four patient identifying factors within the example. The email was not sent securely, nor was it encrypted. Were there any issues with the way that the documentation was sent? If so, what is the BEST way to handle a situation like this?
   a. No issues were found with the scenario. Although PHI was sent unsecured, it was being sent to a work email.
   b. Yes, issues were found with the documentation not being sent securely; however, there was no issue with it being sent to the work email dependent upon the security behind the email traffic and content.
   c. Yes, issues were found with the documentation not being sent securely. It is better to be conservative and send PHI only when necessary and always send securely no matter if the recipient is internal or external.
   d. No issues were found with the scenario. PHI can be sent unencrypted as long as it is sent to the intended recipient for a reasonable and necessary purpose.

60. Release of information has a quick-release functionality in the EHR system that allows the user to release a patient's record at the click of a button. However, there is no way to specify which documentation is to be released, so this functionality submits the patient's entire record each time it is used. There have been no complaints, and productivity is at an all-time high. Based on AHIMA standards, should this functionality continue to be used?
   a. Yes, the process allows the release of information for employees to work more efficiently because records can be released in an instant, increasing productivity.
   b. Yes, with no complaints, it appears that the system is serving its purpose and providing patients with access to their records in a timely manner. Removing the functionality may cause issues with customer service.
   c. There is not enough information to determine whether the functionality is a benefit or detriment to the department.
   d. No, the minimum necessary rule is being violated here because the entire patient record is being sent over, even in the event that only a specific date of service or procedure is being requested.

61. An orthopedic practice incorrectly faxes a patient's records to Hopkins Hospital instead of West Hill Hospital. In following HIPAA guidelines, what should be the next steps taken by the privacy officer?
   a. Document the action as an incident because the incorrect hospital was established as a covered entity.
   b. Document the action as a breach within internal records only.
   c. Document the action as a breach on the HHS site as well as within internal records.
   d. Call and notify/confirm receipt of the documentation by the incorrect facility, request that the documentation be destroyed, and document the action as an incident.

62. It was found that a facility had a 30% error rate involving issues with the transfers of PHI through fax and front-desk handoffs through observation rounds of the facility for a week by the compliance staff. With a problem of this magnitude, which of the following would be the best way to ensure that this is addressed and monitored?
   a. Include this within the risk management initiatives for the year and set up a 3- to 6-month corrective action plan.
   b. Issue company-wide training on the issue and keep a record of the attendees.
   c. Notate the issue and address at a later date; 30% is not enough severity to include in the risk analysis.
   d. Review historical background on the issue, and interview those within areas that were found have the most errors to improve workflow.

63. A laptop from the billing department at Sunflower Medical Center was stolen. The laptop included 478 patients whose PHI was unprotected. The compliance department was notified, and the director of HIM was contacted for a review of the next steps. Which of the following represents the appropriate next steps?

   a. Notification to the patients identified, internal report of the incident, documentation to HHS as an incident, and notification to the media due to the patient counts of PHI being greater than 450 patients.
   b. Notification to the patients identified, internal report of the incident, documentation to HHS as a breach, and notification to the media due to the patient counts of PHI being greater than 450 patients.
   c. Notification to the patients identified, internal report of the incident, and documentation to OCR as a breach. Media notification is not needed due to the patient counts of PHI not exceeding 500 patients.
   d. Notification to the patients identified, internal report of the incident, and documentation to HHS as a breach. Media notification is not needed due to the patient counts of PHI not exceeding 500 patients.

64. On 3/17/19, a patient calls to inform the hospital that she received the record of another patient on 2/21/19. She states that she forgot to notify the hospital; however, as of today, she has shredded the documentation. Would this scenario represent a breach or an incident? What criteria would you use to support your decision?

   a. Incident. The patient notified the hospital within one month of receipt of the incorrect documentation.
   b. Incident. Regardless of timing of the patient notifying the hospital, the patient discarded the information in the proper manner.
   c. Breach. Any notification outside of 1 week within the receipt of incorrect records is considered a breach.
   d. Breach. Although the patient reported the information as well as stated the proper means of discarding the records, she had the information for weeks, and this documentation could have been viewed by anyone.

65. Becca's sister Abby, 15, is scheduled for an appointment at the dental clinic where Becca is working. Becca wanted to know the outcome of her sister's lab visit, so she reviews her record for that date of service. What do you think about Becca's actions?

   a. Becca's actions were reasonable. As her biological sister, she has the ability to review her record with or without Abby's consent because she is a minor.
   b. Becca's actions were reasonable; she is acting within the scope of her role. This is no different than with any other patient.
   c. Becca's actions are improper; she should have treated her sister as she would any other patient and only access charts when necessary.
   d. Becca's actions are improper due to failure to document the review of Abby's chart within the account notes.

66. During an interview with a HIPAA auditor, members of the office personnel of a small chiropractic office stated that all policies and procedures are kept electronically by the compliance officer. All policies are maintained for a minimum 5 years after creation, but they may be updated periodically. With this said, are there any flaws in the office personnel's response?
   a. Yes, policies and procedures should be kept for a minimum of 6 years after the later of the date of the policies' creation and the last effective date. The practice should keep records after the last update to the policies.
   b. Yes, policies and procedures should be kept for a minimum of 5 years after the later of the date of the policies' creation and the last effective date. The practice should keep records after the last update to the policies.
   c. No, the way in which records are handled by the practice is in line with regulation with policies being maintained for a minimum of 5 years.
   d. Yes, policies and procedures should be kept for a minimum of 6 years from the date of creation, regardless of the last effective date or revisions to the policies/procedures.

67. A nurse who is now teaching at a community college uses de-identifiable data in an example for her class. The de-identifiable information included gender, birth month and day, and five-digit ZIP Code. With your knowledge of HIPAA, what is significant, if anything, about this scenario?
   a. The nurse was out of compliance by using the example in her class. Using the patient's birth month and day is not considered de-identifiable and is considered 1 of the 18 identifiers by the HIPAA Privacy Rule.
   b. The nurse was out of compliance by using the example in her class. Using gender in combination with the birth month and day is not considered de-identifiable information.
   c. The nurse was out of compliance by using the example in her class. The use of the five-digit ZIP Code is not considered de-identifiable information.
   d. There is nothing significant about this scenario.

68. Business associate agreements (BAAs) were created out of which of the following?
   a. Clinical Laboratory Improvement Amendments — federal guidelines for all laboratory testing on humans
   b. Health Insurance Portability and Accountability Act (HIPAA) — regulation to modernize the flow of information, protect PHI, and provide limitations on insurance.
   c. Health Information Technology for Economic and Clinical Health (HITECH) Act — addresses privacy and security concerns around the transmission of data.
   d. The Joint Commission — a not-for-profit group that issues voluntary accreditations to healthcare organizations.

69. Within Sunshine Hills Hospital, a patient comes in who has been a victim of domestic violence. An employee immediately calls the police and releases the patient's records to them without the patient's consent. Do you agree or disagree with the employee's actions?
   a. Agree. The employee has the legal right to release the information to the police without consent according to the HIPAA Privacy Rule.
   b. Disagree. The employee has no legal right to release the patient information without the patient's consent according to the HIPAA Privacy Rule.
   c. Disagree. The employee has no legal right to release the patient information without the patient's consent according to the HIPAA Security Rule.
   d. Agree. The employee has the legal right to release the information to the police without consent according to the HIPAA Omnibus Rule.

70. A given EHR system does not allow the customer service team to access progress notes on patients. However, there are a few times when customer service would need to review progress notes, and this use has been approved by senior leadership. In order to execute this, which of the following would yield optimal results while adhering to guidelines?
   a. Creation of an ice-breaker task that allows the user to be required to enter credentials and reasoning as to why access is needed
   b. Request to IT to allow role-based access to progress notes for the customer service team
   c. Creation of a "breaking-the-glass" task that allows the user to be required to enter credentials and reasoning as to why access is needed
   d. Creation of a process called shattering in which the team would be allowed to see a small subset or piece of the progress note, often in a summary format

71. A request is made for the records of a patient with a history of alcohol and drug abuse. The normal release of information workflow is executed by the patient signing a release form. Are there any significant factors that the facility must consider in this scenario?
   a. There is no significance. The normal process of releasing is reasonable with the given scenario.
   b. Due to the patient's history of alcohol and drug abuse, the normal process for releasing information should be followed along with the request being completed in person, review of identification, and notarization of the document.
   c. From the confidentiality perspective, the facility maintaining the record must provide with the disclosure a statement prohibiting redisclosure due to the patient having a history of alcohol and drug abuse.
   d. Due to the sensitive nature of patients with alcohol and drug abuse, patient access is prohibited other than that which has received permission by the provider.

72. Within a hospital emergency room, there are two patients who have the same first and last name (John Smith). In order for the front desk staff to identify the appropriate patient to start the payment process for services rendered, the first and last name of the patient is called along with the patient's birthdate. As a result, several patients within the waiting room have written the hospital to say this was a HIPAA violation. What information can you present for or against the patients' concerns?
   a. This is a HIPAA violation because a patient's first name, last name, and birthdate are patient identifiers. The hospital should discontinue this practice and come up with other ways of identifying patients without the use of identifiers.
   b. This is a HIPAA violation. It would be acceptable to use the patient's first and last name, but in combination with the patient's birthdate this presents an issue. The hospital should discontinue this practice and come up with other ways of identifying patients without the use of identifiers.
   c. This is a HIPAA violation. It would be acceptable to use the patient's birthdate, but in combination with the patient's first and last name this presents an issue. The hospital should discontinue this practice and come up with other ways of identifying patients without the use of identifiers.
   d. This is not a HIPAA violation; although the patient's first name, last name, and birthdate are identifiers, due to the need to use all three to appropriately identify the correct patient for payment purposes, no violation has been made.

73. Steven has been attending Onslow Neurology Clinic since he was 7 years old. Steven, who has turned 18 today, is taken to his appointment by his mother, Ellen. At the conclusion of the appointment, Ellen requests information from the doctor regarding information that was provided to Steven during the appointment. The doctor proceeds to give Ellen a summary of the information given when Steven interrupts stating that his rights have been violated. Is this true?
   a. Yes, his rights have been violated because he is now 18 and therefore has to provide consent for others to hear any information regarding his visit.
   b. No, his rights have not been violated because Ellen is his biological mother; therefore, by law she has a right to receive information regarding his visit.
   c. No, his rights have not been violated because Ellen is the guarantor on the account and is therefore responsible for payment of services, which provides her legal right to her son's information.
   d. No, his rights have not been violated due to fact that this is a neurology patient, and this designation provides a caveat to the normal process of privacy and confidentiality according to HIPAA.

74. A hospital is performing fundraising activities for a local stroke prevention foundation. The foundation has a BAA with the hospital on file. In an effort to aid in fund generation, the hospital agrees to provide patient demographic data, health insurance status, and dates of services without patient authorization. Based on this scenario, what conclusions can be made about the hospital's actions?

a. The hospital will have to self-report to HITECH because the release of patient demographic data, health insurance status, and dates of service is prohibited for fundraising use without patient authorization.
b. The hospital will have to self-report to HHS because the release of patient demographic data, health insurance status, and dates of service is prohibited for fundraising use without patient authorization.
c. The hospital is well within its rights because patient demographic data, health insurance status, and dates of service have been approved for use without patient authorization for fundraising purposes.
d. The hospital will have to self-report to the OCR because the release of patient demographic data, health insurance status, and dates of service is prohibited for fundraising use without patient authorization.

75. A provider is given a new laptop during a facility-wide initiative to update laptops. Her old laptop contains PHI that has been saved to the hard drive. In the process of receiving the new laptop, the provider deletes information from the old laptop and begins use with the new one. What should be the provider's next step?

a. Because PHI items were stored on the hard drive, the provider should keep the laptop just in case information, including PHI, needs to be referenced from it.
b. The provider should give the old laptop to the IT technician for proper wiping/cleaning of the laptop as well as proper disposal of the laptop. Deleting the information stored is not sufficient.
c. The provider should give the old laptop to the HIM department for proper wiping/cleaning of the laptop as well as proper disposal of the laptop. Deleting the information stored is not sufficient.
d. The provider should send the old laptop back to the manufacturer for proper wiping/cleaning of the laptop as well as proper disposal of the laptop. Deleting the information stored is not sufficient.

76. A patient requests seven copies of his medical record. He is told that there will be a $10.00 fee associated with this. The patient threatens to have legal counsel involved because he has a right to access his medical records at any time free of charge according to HIPAA guidelines. The facility disagrees. Are you for or against the patient?

a. For the patient. The patient has a right to receive his medical records timely and without cost according to HIPAA regulations.
b. For the patient. The patient has a right to receive his medical records timely and without cost according to the Stark Law.
c. Against the patient. A facility has the right to charge for any copies in excess of five copies of PHI as long as the associated costs are reasonable.
d. Against the patient. A facility has the right to charge for any copies of PHI as long as the associated costs are reasonable.

77. This is Henry's first visit to the GMK Family Practice facility. At registration, he is given a notice of privacy practices (NPP) form to fill out. Henry refuses to sign the form. With no signature on the form, what effects does this have on the facility?
    a. The facility must inform the patient that he must sign the form because having no documentation of signature could lead to sanctions imposed by HHS.
    b. This does not affect the facility at all; the patient is not required to sign the document, and by law the facility is only required to keep the signed forms on file.
    c. The facility must inform the patient that he must sign the form and that by doing so he is agreeing to any special uses and/or disclosures of his records.
    d. The facility must keep record on file of the patient's refusal to sign the document. This does not affect the provider's ability to use the health information as HIPAA permits.

78. A certified public accounting (CPA) firm is hired by a medical center to provide accounting services. The firm is asked to sign a BAA in which the firm stated that because of the company not performing any repricing information, practice management actions, or utilization review services, a BAA is not required. Are the statements provided by the CPA firm true or false and why?
    a. True, only third parties that provide certain services are required to sign BAAs, and accounting services are not included in those services.
    b. False, accounting services fall under the purview stated within the HIPAA Privacy Rule; therefore, a BAA is needed.
    c. True, the only services in which BAAs are required are repricing information, practice management actions, or utilization review services.
    d. False, accounting services fall under the purview stated within the Medicare Conditions of Participation; therefore, a BA agreement is needed.

79. A subpoena was provided to the HIM department to provide legal health record information for a patient. An HIM employee submitted the request and included statistical reports, incident reports, and quality indicators. Did the HIM employee accurately complete this request?
    a. Although the employee completed the request, the statistical reports, incident reports, and quality indicators should have been omitted because they are not considered as part of the legal health record.
    b. The employee completed the request accurately due to the fact that the legal health record is the patient's record in its entirety, which includes but is not limited to statistical reports, incident reports, and quality indicators.
    c. The employee should have only sent the patient records, statistical reports, and quality indicators. Incident reports are not included in the legal health record.
    d. The employee should have only sent the patient records, incident reports, and quality indicators. Statistical reports are not included in the legal health record.

80. Is a hospital legally permitted to hire a third-party vendor for the disposal of PHI?
    a. Legally, the disposal of records cannot be handed off to a third-party vendor because disposal and accounting for disposal are responsibilities of the hospital.
    b. A third-party vendor is permitted to be hired for the disposal of PHI as long as the total of records disposed monthly does not exceed 500.
    c. A third-party vendor is permitted to be hired for the disposal of PHI as long as the total of records disposed monthly does not exceed 250.
    d. A third-party vendor is permitted to be hired for the disposal of PHI as long as a BAA is in place.

81. The minimum-necessary rule was created to add emphasis on protecting PHI. Does this rule apply for those instances in which the use or disclosure of the information is authorized by the patient?
    a. Yes, the minimum-necessary rule is applicable in all cases regardless of authorization provided by the patient.
    b. No, the minimum-necessary rule is only applicable with the use of information and is not applicable to disclosure of information.
    c. No, the minimum-necessary rule is only applicable with the disclosure of information and is not applicable to the use of information.
    d. No, the minimum-necessary rule does not apply in instances that are authorized by the patient.

82. The HIPAA Security Rule was created to mandate regulation around the electronic and cybersecurity sectors. Is this statement valid?
    a. No, the HIPAA Security Rule includes not only electronic and cybersecurity components but also administrative, technical, and physical safeguard components as well.
    b. Yes, as is stated within the AHIMA standards for security.
    c. Yes, as is stated within the Centers for Medicare & Medicaid Services (CMS) standards for meaningful use.
    d. Yes, as is stated within the CMS standards for Medicare access and CHIP Reauthorization Act/Merit-based Incentive Payment System reporting.

83. The HIM department realizes that John Smith at ABC Hospital has multiple health record numbers. The term used to describe this scenario is which one of the following?
    a. Overlap
    b. Duplicate
    c. Multidimensional account
    d. Overlay

84. The _____ is the committee responsible for protecting the rights of human research studies who participate in research activities.
    a. Joint Commission
    b. Officer of Inspector General
    c. Institutional Review Board
    d. Office of Civil Rights

85. In the example SELECT patient name FROM patients WHERE gender = m, which term describes what data to get?
   a. SELECT
   b. FROM
   c. WHERE
   d. All of the above

86. Within a data model, the current format of the patient's admit date is as follows: DD_MM_YY. However, the agreed-upon format was determined to be DD_MM_YYYY. To accurately display the agreed-upon format, at which level does the change need to occur?
   a. Schema
   b. Table
   c. Data dictionary
   d. Query

87. Phases of the systems development life cycle (SDLC) include which of the following?
   a. Planning, scope, design, and implementation
   b. Scope, critical pathway, planning, and analysis
   c. Planning, analysis, design, and implementation
   d. Planning, analysis, critical pathway, and implementation

88. Which quality management function performs the evaluation of medical necessity and effective and efficient use of healthcare services and procedures?
   a. Clinical quality management
   b. Utilization management
   c. Risk management
   d. Operational efficiency management

89. _____ events are monitored by the Joint Commission and are defined as events that are unforeseen within the healthcare setting that lead to death or injury (physical or psychological).
   a. Sentinel
   b. Morbidity
   c. Sepsis
   d. Miscellaneous

90. Tina's manager asked her to calculate the range of length-of-stay (LOS) days in the month of August in FY19. In order to do this, Tina must do which of the following?
   a. Subtract the lowest number of LOS days from the highest number of LOS days.
   b. Add up all LOS days and divide by the total days in the month of August.
   c. Report the number of LOS days that is most frequent in August.
   d. Report all LOS days in FY19 and compare those days to the LOS days in FY18.

91. Healthcare information systems' ability to communicate and work with each other in different organizations, demographic areas, and settings is defined as which one of the following?

    a. Interface management
    b. Telemedicine
    c. Personal health records (PHRs)
    d. Interoperability

92. Which one of the following presents the most secure way of communicating with a patient in regard to their questions, issues, and concerns with a given health provider?

    a. Email
    b. PHR
    c. Patient portal
    d. Text message

93. Which of the following is an example of data security?

    a. Saving patient information containing PHI to a hard drive
    b. Sending patient test results through the hospital's email to the email address provided by the patient
    c. The use of encryption during the saving and transmission of data
    d. Performing telemedicine

94. Which one of the following is a common form of network consisting of a central switch acting as the transmission administrator to send messages and providing a common point for nodes within the network?

    a. Bus topology
    b. Train topology
    c. Star topology
    d. Hexagonal topology

95. End-user feedback in regard to user needs and expectations of information is best gathered using which one of the following?

    a. IT ticket request
    b. Questionnaires
    c. Monitored workflow
    d. Statistics

96. Which of the following is used by CMS to access the need of prepayment audits for a given healthcare provider?

    a. Predictive modeling
    b. Statistical sampling
    c. Current-year reporting analysis
    d. Bell curve review

97. All of the following prohibit interoperability and or health information exchange EXCEPT which one of the following?
   a. Hybrid record keeping
   b. Complete use of EHR systems by all communicating facilities
   c. System disconnections
   d. Lack of standardization

98. A facility has portable devices that are not locked up when not in use. The facility also does not keep track of the portable devices. Which security component would this vulnerability fall under?
   a. Administrative safeguards
   b. Physical safeguards
   c. Technical safeguards
   d. Organizational safeguards

99. Patients are required to be notified about the facility's use of their PHI as well as their rights in regard to their PHI. What is this called?
   a. Privacy and security policy
   b. Notice of privacy practices (NPP)
   c. Business associate agreement
   d. Medical records release

100. Health information interoperability goes hand in hand with which of the following?
   a. Demographic availability to personal health records (PHRs)
   b. Comprehensive and complete public standards
   c. Data mining and analysis
   d. Laws governing medical record release

101. Parkview Hospital has called upon its business analyst to complete an analysis on the strength of the relationship between high blood pressure and stroke within a certain patient population. Which of the following statistical tools would be the best one to address the needs of the hospital?
   a. Predictive modeling
   b. Frequency distribution
   c. Z-score determination
   d. Linear regression

102. The pharmacy department has acquired new software changing the way that work flows and information exchange occurs in the department. For the purposes of data tracking, which of the following would also need to be updated?
   a. Data flow diagram
   b. Facility organizational chart
   c. The selected schema
   d. Data dictionary

103. Delinquent records are limited to _____, as set by the Joint Commission. If this is exceeded, there will be consequences imposed by the Joint Commission.
   a. 15% of monthly discharges
   b. 50% of the average number of admissions
   c. 50% of the average number of discharges
   d. 50% of the average LOSs in the current month

104. Within informatics, which of the following is used to identify future trends and patterns based on the previous analysis of behavior?
   a. Algorithms
   b. Standard deviation
   c. Linear regression
   d. Quantitative research

105. The develop phase of SDLC includes which of the following?
   a. Marketing, installation and configuration of code, and graphic design
   b. Installation, configuration, writing, and testing of code
   c. Marketing, installation and configuration of code, and administration of training
   d. Writing and testing of code, scheduling of projects, and graphic design

106. Bryant Hospital experienced a power outage due to a natural disaster. This caused data to be lost throughout the healthcare system after a system failure. However, the hospital was able to retrieve lost data through which of the following?
   a. Data recovery
   b. Data backup
   c. Data mining
   d. Data warehousing

107. Which of the following represents correct terminal-digit ordering?
   a. 01-28-32, 24-47-26, 18-52-12
   b. 01-28-32, 24-47-43, 18-52-56
   c. 01-28-30, 24-52-29, 18-47-29
   d. 01-30-15, 24-15-07, 18-18-18

108. Prepayment audits performed by CMS are selected with the use of predictive modeling. To ensure that the selected samples are without bias, CMS may use which sampling tool?
   a. Random sampling
   b. Basic algorithms
   c. Bell-curve review
   d. Stratified sampling

109. Which of the following is true regarding personal health records (PHRs)?
   a. PHRs are controlled by the provider; patients have view-only access.
   b. Patients and provider determine access rights.
   c. PHRs allow individuals to manage and own their own record.
   d. Giving patients access to their PHRs has been found to provide no impact on patient health outcomes.

110. Healthcare facilities are placing more emphasis on electronic information and telecommunications to aid in patient care. This has now been defined as:
   a. E-Health
   b. E-Communication
   c. Digital care
   d. Telehealth

111. Which data would be best represented by a pie chart?
   a. The number of patients discharged by department
   b. A comparison of sepsis cases over the past 6 months
   c. The number of audits performed per hospital department
   d. Percentages of major hand-off risk factors in the pharmacy department

112. Grover Healthcare System is implementing a new EHR system. In order to make sure that issues and problems are tracked in a way in which they can be reviewed and accessed timely, what should the organization have in place?
   a. An issues-management program/protocol
   b. A satisfaction survey
   c. Periodic feedback sessions
   d. A manual department log of incidents

113. Within consumer informatics, the objective is to achieve which of the following?
   a. Increase consumer use of PHRs.
   b. Aid in the consumer's engagement with their healthcare providers.
   c. Increase patient health literacy, education, and patient-focused informatics.
   d. Provide marketing data to healthcare providers to strengthen consumer relationships through their experiences with their patients.

114. You are an associate vice president at PJ Hospital. The radiology department is interested in developing new workflows around their processes and the way in which they transmit their imaging. As the director, you want to verify the standards associated with this process. Which standard best addresses the needs of the radiology department?
   a. HL7
   b. SNOWMED CT
   c. DICOM
   d. LOINC

115. Within conceptual data modeling, reviewing the instances in which one entity is associated with another involves which concept?
   a. Cardinality
   b. Defining relationships
   c. Composite attributes
   d. Optional attributes

116. In 2013, two hospitals, Hospital A and Hospital B, implemented the same EHR system. Hospital A had a plan to implement the EHR in the clinics first, the north side of the hospital second, and the south side of the hospital third. Hospital B chose to implement all departments on the same day at the same time. Which process did each hospital take with implementation?

    a. Hospital A took the domino approach, and Hospital B took the straight-line approach.
    b. Hospital A took the phased rollout approach, and Hospital B took the big-bang approach.
    c. Hospital A took the domino approach, and Hospital B took the big-bang approach.
    d. Hospital A took the phased rollout approach, and Hospital B took the straight-line approach.

117. The HIM department reports on issues with documentation, LOS, and coding. According to regulations, a facility is to report on delinquency and notify the appropriate regulatory body. In this case, the regulatory body to report the delinquency to would be which one of the following?

    a. OCR — Delinquency would be reported here because it governs civil rights and HIPAA issues.
    b. Institutional review board — Delinquency would be reported here because it involves clinical research subjects and their rights.
    c. Joint Commission — Delinquency would be reported here because this information is needed to make important decision about the facility's ability to provide quality care.
    d. AHIMA — Delinquency would be reported here because the concept of delinquency was founded here and is reported out through this organization for awareness.

118. A physician provides a verbal order to a technician to perform three tests on a particular patient. This order is not documented in the EHR system. Upon auditor review, progress notes indicate that testing was performed by the technician but there was no documentation to show that the test given to the patient was the test that the physician requested. From the HIM perspective, which of the following should happen?

    a. A conversation with the department to ensure that this does not happen again. No further changes are required to documentation within the EHR.
    b. Nothing needs to happen, if the provider signs the technician document of test that was received, this is sufficient data to support the test performed.
    c. Recommendation from HIM that the technician no longer performs testing.
    d. A conversation with the department, EHR systems team, and HIM to make sure that orders from the physician are documented within the EHR, that the staff is aware of this going forward as is taught/trained to do so, and that they follow up to ensure this was carried out appropriately.

119. A business analyst is asked to pull data on possible correlations between the patient age and their readmission rates for the neurology department. The data should be shown by an executive summary and a graphical depiction. From the graphical perspective, what graph would best convey the needs of the department?

    a. Contingency table
    b. Histogram
    c. Bar graph
    d. Bell curve

120. LA Hospital wants to review their gross death rate for the month of August. The hospital had 15 reported deaths and 1,000 discharges in total, 750 of which did not include infants. What was the hospital's gross death rate for the month of August?

- a. 2%
- b. 20%
- c. 1.5%
- d. 15%

121. The pharmacy wants to ensure that the right medications are given to the right patient and that the system reflects this in a timely manner. Workflows have now been in place for the patient to receive medications at the bedside, and this is scanned into the EHR. In order for this to work as planned, which informatics component is involved?

- a. Bar coding
- b. Topology
- c. Master data file
- d. Optical character recognition

122. The HIM coding department is reviewing data for coding edits due to medical necessity. They find that the coders have been using an outdated local coverage determination (LCD) loaded into the system that has resulted in several claims being billed out incorrectly. What scenario below represents the best way to handle this issue?

- a. Document the encounter on the issues list for informatics, have the outdated LCD removed, consult the billing team for correction, conduct monitoring through the EHR system that claims have been sent out to payers correctly, and educate staff.
- b. Document the issue and notify billing of the change to go forward as of today, but no retrospective action is needed.
- c. Only the removal of the outdated LCD is needed.
- d. Only training of the HIM staff is needed.

123. With promotion of interoperability through the use of EHRs, how could one judge the accuracy of a given EHR system with this in mind?

- a. Accuracy can be judged by how well the system coincides with Joint Commission regulations and standards.
- b. Reviewing how well the EHR system performed during meaningful use reviews performed by CMS.
- c. Reviewing how well the EHR system has clear standards on terminology, content/formatting, data transport, and how they stack up to national requirements.
- d. Accuracy of interoperability cannot be determined without research of two or more facilities that use EHRs to determine how well they would communicate and transmit information between each other should a patient be seen in all facilities.

124. Hospital A has several data elements that are defined through a data dictionary. Hospital B has several data elements but no formal data dictionary. From the perspective of interoperability, does this help or hinder the overall interoperability goals?

   a. This hinders interoperability in that although Hospital A has a data dictionary in which the meaning for data elements can be derived, Hospital B leaves the meaning of data elements up to interpretation by the user.
   b. This aids interoperability because it promotes communication between the two facilities to understand the associated data elements and provide an opportunity for suggestions/recommendations for the process.
   c. This hinders interoperability because in order for it to be achieved, both hospitals need the same data elements and data dictionary.
   d. This neither aids nor hinders interoperability because data dictionaries are not a requirement for interoperability to be achieved.

125. A research study was developed to test that patient no-show encounters in family medicine clinic are higher during morning appointments than they are in afternoon appointments. Which of the following statements would be suitable within the analysis report and why?

   a. The alternative hypothesis would be that no-show encounters are higher during afternoon appointments. This is because the alternative hypothesis represents the opposite of the original hypothesis.
   b. The null hypothesis would be that no-show encounters are higher during morning appointments. This is because the null hypothesis represents what coincides with the original hypothesis.
   c. In this scenario, there is no need for an alternative or null hypothesis because the original hypothesis can be easily proven through data.
   d. The null hypothesis would be that no-show encounters are not statistically different between morning and afternoon appointments. This is because the null hypothesis represents the idea that differences in observed data are solely the result of random chance.

126. What are the differences in functional and process interoperability?

   a. Functional interoperability is one step below process interoperability. Functional interoperability is the successful transmission or receipt of data. Process interoperability is taking data that are transmitted and received to create data sets.
   b. This question cannot be answered because "functional" is not a type of interoperability.
   c. This question cannot be answered because "process" is not a type of interoperability.
   d. Process interoperability is one step below process interoperability. Process interoperability is the transmission or receipt of data successfully. Functional interoperability is taking data that are transmitted and received to create data sets.

127. Which of the following is an example of an advantage of structured query language?

   a. Easy user access
   b. Full control of the database
   c. Well-defined standards
   d. Low operating cost

128. Smithfield Hospital wants to acquire a new EHR system. The hospital has several onsite product demonstrations to ensure that the capabilities of the system are a good match to its needs and to promote buy-in with all stakeholders. Contract negotiation has taken place, and the budget for this initiative has been approved by the hospital's chief financial officer. Are the above-mentioned items enough to support due diligence?
   a. Yes, onsite project demonstrations, contract negotiating, and budget approval are enough to support due diligence.
   b. No, additional items such as time frame of experience in the field should be considered to prove due diligence.
   c. No, additional items such as credit and reference checks should be considered to prove due diligence.
   d. No, additional items such as customer satisfaction of various departments within the vendor should be considered to prove due diligence.

129. A review of statistical data showed that the more education that patients are given on site, the better their outcomes tend to be. What conclusions can you draw from this statement?
   a. Patient education and patient outcomes are positively correlated.
   b. Patient education and patient outcomes are negatively correlated.
   c. There is no correlation between patient education and patient outcomes.
   d. More information is needed to determine if a correlation exists.

130. A hospital administrator asks you which is the better measure to use when reviewing LOS: the average or the range. Which answer would you provide and why?
   a. The average LOS because the average provides the most accurate depiction of what is happening.
   b. The range LOS because it accounts for the extreme "outliers" within the data.
   c. Neither average nor range LOS should be used for measurement.
   d. The average LOS because it accounts for the extreme "outliers" within the data.

131. Within a healthcare setting, the clinical documentation improvement (CDI) team helps to support coders as well as providers to avoid:
   a. Local code determination issues
   b. Assumption coding
   c. Medically unlikely edits (MUEs)
   d. National Correct Coding Initiative (NCCI) edits

132. Margot is a coder for Sunnyville Hospital. She notices that a combination code is available for the procedure that she is reviewing, but she knows that if she breaks the combination code into two separate codes, she can achieve higher reimbursement. This is an example of which of the following?
   a. Multitier coding
   b. Undercoding
   c. Upcoding
   d. Unbundling

133. Which program was developed with the purpose of the reduction and prevention of improper billing payments with respect to Medicare claims?
    a. The False Claims Act
    b. The Joint Commission
    c. The Recovery Audit Contractor program
    d. The HITECH Act

134. A document that a patient signed prior to treatment for a service that has been deemed to likely not be paid by Medicare that outlines the type of service, reason for possible noncoverage by Medicare, as well as the estimated associated costs is called a/an _____. This document also states that the patient will be liable for the estimated cost listed if Medicare does not pay the claim.
    a. ABN
    b. MSP
    c. ERM
    d. EOB

135. When reviewing a facility's accounts receivable, the standard increment used to represent the aging of accounts is the:
    a. 90-day increment
    b. 30-day increment
    c. 15-day increment
    d. 20-day increment

136. A request for payment sent from a facility to an insurance company is an example of a/an:
    a. Contractual adjustment
    b. Allowance
    c. Revenue recognition
    d. Claim

137. Several patients at Mint Hill Hospital have suspected breaches of their personal information during a recent hospital stay. Per HIPAA policy, these violations should be reported to:
    a. the Department of Health and Human Services through the Office of Inspector General (OIG) within 100 days of the violation.
    b. the CMS within 90 days of the violation.
    c. the Department of Health and Human Services through the Office for Civil Rights (OCR) within 180 days of the violation.
    d. the Joint Commission within 60 days of the violation.

138. Medical identity theft violations are reported to which agency?
    a. Office of Civil Rights
    b. Office of Inspector General
    c. HHS
    d. Internal Revenue Service

139. _____ is an important component of the prearrival/front-end process for scheduled patients.
   a. Charge capture
   b. Charge description master (CDM) management
   c. Clinical documentation
   d. Insurance verification

140. Coding compliance is a key element within the healthcare setting. Ongoing coding compliance education should include all of the following EXCEPT:
   a. OIG work plans
   b. International Classification of Diseases, Tenth Revision, Clinical Modification (ICD-10 CM), and ICD-Procedure Coding System (PCS) guidelines
   c. Previous years' updates to the ICD-10, Current Procedural Terminology (CPT), and Healthcare Common Procedures Coding System (HCPCS) coding systems
   d. Changes in reimbursement systems

141. Which government-sponsored program provides healthcare coverage to low-income individuals?
   a. Medicare
   b. Medicaid
   c. TRICARE
   d. None of the above

142. Paul Newman has an insurance plan in which he can only go to certain doctors, other healthcare providers, or facilities that are on the plan's list besides emergency services. Paul has which of the following types of plan?
   a. Special needs
   b. Preferred provider organization (PPO)
   c. Health maintenance organization (HMO)
   d. Private health

143. Amber goes to her neurologist's office and learns that the facility was unable to determine which insurance listed for Amber is the primary insurance and which one is secondary. Receiving this information will ensure that no duplication of benefits will be paid. What type of issue is this?
   a. EOB
   b. Coordination of benefits
   c. Medicare summary notice
   d. Remittance advice

144. Lullah is told that she will need an MRI by her doctor. Per her insurance, the physician's office needs to obtain permission to go forth with services if the facility wants insurance to pay for the procedure. This is called which one of the following?
   a. Financial counseling
   b. Insurance eligibility
   c. Preauthorization
   d. Benefits review

145. In an effort for Jordan Hospital to review the cost of providing care to its patients to its diagnosis-related group mix of patients in relation to other hospitals, which coding element should the hospital be reviewing?
   a. LOS days
   b. Case-mix index
   c. Total days in AR
   d. Days in total discharged, not final billed (DNFB)

146. Common denial reasons include all of the following EXCEPT:
   a. Noncovered services
   b. Lack of medical necessity
   c. Lack of preauthorization
   d. Removal of modifiers when found to be unnecessary

147. Those individuals who are found to have been acting in a fraudulent, wasteful, and/or abusive manner when receiving payments from the government can be:
   a. Found in violation of the False Claims Act
   b. Found in violation of the Deficit Reduction Act of 2005
   c. Excluded from being allowed to participate in federal programs
   d. Found in violation of HIPAA

148. Sunnyville Family Practice has been found to be in violation of the False Claims Act. Medicare is applying the error rate across claims within the last 3 years as a correction of payment. What is this process called?
   a. Target area review
   b. Extrapolation
   c. Observation
   d. Zone Program Integrity Contractor review

149. Clinical documentation improvement (CDI) and _____ work together to educate medical staff members on documentation requirements.
   a. compliance
   b. hospital billing
   c. HIM
   d. the charge data master team

150. Once the hospital coding team codes a claim and it is considered complete, many facilities have an auditing system called a/an _____ built into their EHRs to place the claim against edits to aid in the clean-claim process.
   a. NCCI edit
   b. charge data master
   c. claim scrubber
   d. EOB

151. Typically, "days" in accounts receivable start at the:
   a. Date of admission
   b. Date of discharge
   c. Date the claim is received by the payer
   d. Date the claim is billed

152. What is the name of the healthcare program geared toward supporting active-duty military and other eligible members?

   a. TRICARE
   b. Medicare
   c. Medicaid
   d. Commercial insurance

153. What is the methodology that places the quality of patient care as a priority and provides incentives and penalties depending on the meeting of certain measures?

   a. Fee for service
   b. Capitation
   c. Value-based care
   d. Diagnosis-related groups

154. A request for payment from a healthcare facility to an insurance provider is considered a/an:

   a. Reimbursement
   b. Allowance
   c. Contractual adjustment
   d. Claim

155. A denial report was created for the pediatric department. The report showed the following denial sources: authorization denials, registration denials, billing denials, and non-covered-service denials. Out of the sources listed, which are considered avoidable denials?

   a. Avoidable denials would be represented by authorization and registration denials.
   b. Registration denials are the only denials in this scenario that are considered avoidable.
   c. None of the listed denials are considered avoidable denials.
   d. All of the listed denials are considered avoidable denials.

156. Accounts receivable reported is reviewed by key stakeholders and is shown to have been down 10% from the last quarter. What does this mean?

   a. The time frame from the patient's discharge date to the receipt of payment has improved by 10%.
   b. The time frame from when the payer receives the claim to when the payment is received by the facility has improved by 10%.
   c. The time frame from the date that the claim was billed to the receipt of payment has improved by 10%.
   d. The time frame from the patient's admission date to the receipt of payment has declined by 10%.

157. _____ aid in determining the value of a data governance program and are sometimes called success measures.

   a. Goals
   b. Controls
   c. Mission statements
   d. Key performance indicators

158. A description of an organizations future goals and optimal state is outlined in the organization's:
   a. Vision statement
   b. Mission statement
   c. Strategic plan
   d. SMART goals

159. Self-awareness, self-regulation, motivation, empathy, and social skills are all attributes of:
   a. Role theory
   b. Interpersonal activity
   c. Decisional activity
   d. Emotional intelligence

160. Pierre is a part of a healthcare organization that is transitioning to a new EHR system. Although he is not eager to try the new system, Pierre has witnessed management's activities and views on the new system and is comfortable and willing to accept the new system. Pierre is a part of which group?
   a. Innovators
   b. Early adopters
   c. Early majority
   d. Late majority

161. A description of an organization's purpose for existing is:
   a. Vision statement
   b. Mission statement
   c. Strategic plan
   d. A SMART goal

162. Which of the following types of graphical representations identifies the beginning and completion of work projects and illustrates any scheduling overlaps and miscalculations.
   a. Gantt chart
   b. Box plot
   c. Pie chart
   d. Bar graph

163. A terminally ill patient has refused any treatment for his cancer. This is an example of which of the following ethical principles?
   a. Beneficence
   b. Altruism
   c. Autonomy
   d. Egoism

164. AHIMA's Code of Ethics encompasses professional core values that include which of the following?
   a. Communication, integrity, respect, and quality
   b. Leadership, quality, respect, and integrity
   c. Integrity, communication, equality, and respect
   d. Integrity, leadership, quality, and communication

165. The AHIMA Code of Ethics illustrates/serves how many purposes?
 a. 7
 b. 4
 c. 5
 d. 10

166. HIM professionals' ethical obligations extend to:
 a. Patients
 b. The healthcare profession
 c. The public
 d. All of the above

167. Complete positions/job descriptions contain:
 a. Ways to contact the hiring manager
 b. Qualifications needed to effectively perform the job
 c. Salary ranges
 d. Promotional opportunities

168. Documented skills/abilities, knowledge, and characteristics needed in an individual define a:
 a. Job specification
 b. Job description
 c. Position standard
 d. 30- 60-, and 90-day plans

169. The conflict management principle that requires all parties included to let go or give up a piece of their position or responsibilities is considered:
 a. Control
 b. Compromise
 c. Constructive confrontation
 d. Mediation

170. All of the following are true with regard to professional coaching EXCEPT:
 a. Coaching starts with the onboarding of new employees and is evoked as a continuous process.
 b. Coaching involves only teaching and advice components.
 c. Correcting performance issues and improving moral foundation are functions of coaching.
 d. Mentoring is a form of coaching.

171. How does mentoring differ from coaching?
 a. Mentoring is normally conducted on a one-to-one basis.
 b. Knowledge shared/provided by the mentor is primarily focused on current advancement.
 c. Knowledge shared/provided by the mentor is primarily focused on past achievements.
 d. None of the above; mentoring and coaching are one and the same.

172. Effective work standards include the notion that the standard can be met without the cost outweighing the benefit or value of having the standard. This defines which one of the following effective standards?

a. Equitable
b. Attainable
c. Significant
d. Economical

173. Mike has been given the task to provide analysis on how quickly the facility can turn its assets into cash. Which ratio(s) would provide the best solution?

a. Return on investment
b. Current ratio
c. Total margin ratio
d. All of the above

174. Evan has assisted Cruz Hospital in establishing controls that find issues with claims presenting with the incorrect diagnosis. Which of the following has Evan created?

a. Corrective control
b. Preventive control
c. Detective control
d. Avoidable control

175. In 2017, Christian Medical Center had the following report:

	August			September	
Department Supplies:	Budget	Actual	Department Revenue:	Budget	Actual
	$600	$900		$800	$975

Which of the following is correct with regard to variance analysis?

a. August, unfavorable; September, favorable
b. August, unfavorable; September, unfavorable
c. August, favorable; September, favorable
d. August, favorable; September, unfavorable

176. The fax machine within the HIM department needs repairing at least once a month. The director of HIM conducts an analysis in which he finds that it cost $250 to fix the existing machine resulting in a $3,000 expense per year. To purchase a new machine with a 10-year warranty that covers repairs in full, the cost is $2,000. Which type of analysis is the best depiction of the above scenario?

a. Expense analysis
b. Root-cause analysis
c. Cost–benefit analysis
d. Variance analysis

177. The time required to recoup the cost of an investment is considered the:

a. Payback period
b. Opportunity cost
c. Profit period
d. Rate of return

178. Ally decides that she wants to be an organ donor, to help anyone who can benefit from her organs. Which ethical principle does this support?
- a. Beneficence
- b. Least harm
- c. Utilitarianism
- d. Deontology

179. The minimum-necessary concept that states that information should only be viewed by those authorized to do so while only reviewing what is necessary to complete the task at hand is called:
- a. Blanket authorization
- b. Need to know
- c. Authorization review
- d. Release of information

180. All of the following are considered internal environmental assessments EXCEPT:
- a. Financial performance
- b. Performance indicators
- c. Role statements and organizational framework
- d. Competitor analysis

Answer Key and Explanations for Test #1

1. D: Excludes 2 means "not included here." This means that the condition excluded is not a part of the condition represented by the code; however, a patient may have both conditions at the same time. The term see indicates that the coder must seek or refer to an alternate term. Excludes 1 means "not coded here." This means that the excluded condition should never be coded at the same time as the condition represented by the code. The term code also means that two codes may be used to fully describe the condition.

2. A: Although the total number of records, how and where the records will be obtained (medium), and the cost associated with record retention all play a part in the decision-making process, the first and primary concern of record retention is to review state and federal laws and regulations to ensure that records are maintained for the longest time required.

3. B: According to 42 CFR § 482.24, the hospital must maintain a medical record for each inpatient and outpatient encounter. Medical records must be retained in their original or legally reproduced form for a period of at least 5 years.

4. C: SNOWMED CT is a standardized, multilingual vocabulary of clinical terminology used by healthcare providers for the exchange of clinical health information electronically. MEDCIN is a clinical terminology with a strong focus on the facilitation of documentation by providing choices that are in line with providers' clinical thought processes. The National Drug Code (NDC) is the universal product identifier for human drugs.

5. A: Primary data are data that were documented by the healthcare professionals who provided care, treatment, and services for the patient. Aggregate data are data on groups of people that do not identity the patients individually. An index is a report from a database that allows for the location of diagnoses, procedures, physicians, etc. to be found within the database.

6. C: Based on the fact that the question mentions neoplasms as well as stage and site, cancer is the correct answer choice. Diabetes, immunization, and trauma registries do not address the criteria, nor do they serve the purpose of diagnosing and treating cancer.

7. A: The American National Standards Institute (ANSI) is responsible for creating standards to address healthcare transactions between health partners. The American Society for Testing and Material (ASTM) is responsible for creating standards with regard to the EHR. Health Level-7 (HL7) is responsible for creating standards in regard to the content of the EHR. The Outcome and Assessment Information Set (OASIS) is a data set that is associated with the home health prospective payment system.

8. B: Unstructured data provide the user the opportunity to review detailed data in its granularity. This cannot be done with structured data.

9. A: Root operation release means "freeing a body part from an abnormal physical contract by cutting or force." Detachment means "cutting off all or part of the upper or lower extremities." Destruction means "physical eradication of all or a portion of a body part by the direct use of energy, force, or a destructive agent."

10. B: The freeing of a body part from an abnormal physical contract by cutting or force corresponding root operation is called release. The taking or cutting out of solid matter from a body part corresponding root operation is called extirpation. The taking or letting out of fluids and/or gases from a body part corresponding root operation is called drainage.

11. B: The cutting off without replacement corresponding root operation is excision. Cutting off with replacement has no root operation associated. The breaking solid matter into pieces corresponding root operation is fragmentation.

12. A: Encrypting is an appropriate format for electronic format. Burning is not a feasible way of destroying. Although burning could take place, it is not the most appropriate method. Placing information in a locked drawer away from patient access is not destroying data.

13. B: Disaster recovery plans usually involve getting systems up and running after a disaster takes place. Examples include information technology (IT) infrastructure and accessing files offsite. Training is conducted with employees on the business continuity plan itself. Risk and audit controls are not relevant to natural disaster situations; these processes are implemented and enforced regarding normal business practices.

14. C: The Affordable Care Act required most United States citizens to have healthcare coverage. The Omnibus Budget Reconciliation Act mandated the development of a prospective system for hospital-based outpatient services to Medicare beneficiaries. The HITECH Act focused on adoption of IT in health care through economic incentives.

15. A: Identifying and resolving quality issues are functions of data governance for information intelligence. Establishing a risk management program, implementing security awareness for employees, and facility data security planning are all elements of data governance in relation to data quality management.

16. D: Data security management creates policies and procedures to protect security from a compliance and regulatory standpoint. Terminology and classification management involves healthcare technologies, data sets, and classification systems that a facility may use. Content management includes managing structured and unstructured data.

17. B: Open-record review is the review of records while the patient is currently within the facility or while the patient is receiving active treatment. Discharged patient and retro-quality reviews are not terms used within HIM.

18. B: IEEE is an organization that developed the standards for abbreviated test language. ADA are those standards set for those with disabilities. ISO standards are international standards composed of various national standards organizations.

19. A: Schema mapping is the process by which entity relationship diagrams are converted into tables. Attributes are the characteristics within an entity relationship diagram. Normalization is the process that eliminates errors associated with updates, deletions etc., of data within a database.

20. C: The consistency principle is the need for data to be consistent and reliable. Precision speaks to how close to an actual numerical value a measurement is. Granularity consists of the individual data components that cannot be divided further. Timeliness is the concept around receiving information when needed in a timely manner.

21. C: Hydrocephalus in a newborn relates to a defect at birth. The other registries are not applicable in this case.

22. D: Progress notes should be completed by the provider. Administrators, HIM professionals, and registration staff should not have access to amend, delete, or alter a progress note in any way.

23. B: Although all of the answer choices are considered legal documents, only the durable power of attorney is able to act on behalf of the patient in the described circumstances.

24. A: Accreditation standards dictate those standards and rules in regard to the retention and destruction of healthcare information. While HIPAA rules contain some specific retention requirements, it is important to note the distinction between HIPAA records and PHI itself. HIPAA records are those that facilities must maintain to demonstrate HIPAA compliance. HIPAA rules only cover HIPAA record retention.

25. D: Although the actions of coders may ultimately maximize reimbursement, they may result in decreased write-offs and claim edit hold-ups by issuing clean claims. The overall focus of certified coders is to ensure that each claim is coded with accuracy and precision.

26. B: Financial data includes information about the patient's insurance, occupation, and employer. Demographic data include data involving the patient's address, name, date of birth, etc. Accreditation data are not related to the patient but to the standards carried out by the organization. Patient/disease registries are considered clinical data.

27. C: Data mining includes finding patterns and trends within large data sets. Data analysis is modeling data with the intent of meeting a goal or to support decision making within an organization. A data dictionary analysis is a review of the standards and meanings of data within a system.

28. D: Dilation is the enlargement of a tubular body part or orifice. Fragmentation is a procedure that involves breaking solid matter into pieces. Occlusion is completely closing an orifice or the lumen of a tubular body part.

29. C: Although creating proper documentation and maintaining records can at times aid in the receipt of reimbursement, help to avoid malpractice issues, and help in following guidelines, the overall goal is to aid in the continuity of care for all patients.

30. C: Source-oriented records are recognized according to the source. Problem-oriented medical records involve the problem list being the focal point because it is the table of contents for the records. Ascending health records are not a part of HIM terminology.

31. D: Patient identifiers are considered to be part of the financial data category, whereas all of the other answer choices are considered to be clinical data.

32. B: The board of directors consists of elected members who work together with the chief executive officer to develop a hospital's strategic direction. The chief nursing officer and chief information officer serve as administrative staff in support of the chief executive officer.

33. A: Constitutional law is written law and is considered the highest law of the land and takes precedence over state and local laws. Administrative law is written law that controls a government agency or administrative operations. Statutory law is written law established by federal and state legislatures.

34. D: Although the patient has rights to their health records, the record itself actually belongs to the organization that created and maintained the physical record.

35. A: Information governance involves the oversight of data outputs. Data quality is reviewing data to review its quality level based on the goal or parameter set. Data enterprise management is the process of defining, integrating, and retrieving data for internal and external communication.

36. B: Data governance involves the oversight of data inputs. Data quality management involves reviewing data to review their quality level based on the goal or parameter set. Data enterprise management is the process of defining, integrating, and retrieving data for internal and external communication.

37. A: When more than 500 individuals have been affected by a breach, this requires that the media as well as HHS be notified. Anything less than 500 requires notification only to HHS.

38. B: The terms nonrequired, mandatory, and tentative are not associated with the content within the HIPAA Security Rule.

39. B: Technical safeguards are those safeguards that involve the protection of access and control of electronic protected health information (ePHI). Administrative safeguards are put forth to manage actions, policies, and procedures to detect and correct violations. Physical safeguards are used to identify measures to protect systems and equipment, such as identification badges, from natural and environmental hazards. Organizational safeguards include arrangements made between organizations to protect ePHI, such as BAAs.

40. A: When federal and state laws conflict, the body of law that is most stringent is what should be followed.

41. B: Gender is not considered to be an identifier within the HIPAA Privacy Rule.

42. C: The Healthcare Quality Improvement Act was enacted in 1986 as a response to the increasingly high number of malpractice cases in the previous decade to serve as a mitigation attempt. The act included standards or peer reviews by providers.

43. B: Pareto charts are most helpful when reviewing data that contain different categories with a focus on frequency. Flowcharts are best used when documenting current processes. Bar graphs are optimal when reviewing data changes over long periods of time.

44. A: A principal investigator performed due diligence by having the study participant sign the informed consent form. This form is required by HIPAA. For research purposes, it must contain elements outlined by HIPAA guidelines. This question scenario assumed that this requirement is met.

45. C: The Stark Law states that a physician may not refer a patient to a facility in which he or she has financial interest including ownership, compensation agreements, and/or investments.

46. B: The length of time specified for maintaining records may vary from facility to facility.

47. D: Patient incompetency is one exception to the written authorization rule provided by the patient; however, legal documentation has to be presented to a facility in order to be fully compliant with medical record release.

48. B: Although most states adhere to the majority age being 18 and older, there are states in which this is not true. It is important to validate this in cases in which the age of majority is a determining factor in decision making.

49. A: Biological parents of children each have equal rights to medical decision-making as well as release of information on their children, unless there is a court document stating otherwise. One parent may not exclude the other without this document.

50. C: There is no documentation supporting the other answer choices in reference to the exact locations of NPPs, timing or receipt to patients, or the medium in which the document must be received.

51. C: Although both facilities may participate in contracts with managed care, the fact that they are governed by HIPAA makes them covered entities in the eyes of the law. Regulated parties and third-party covered agents are not terms within HIM.

52. A: A threat would be something likely to cause damage or harm. Although this is not an ideal situation for the facility, in its current state, there is no harm done. Although the vulnerability could become a potential breach or incident, there is no action within the scenario that fits the characteristics of either of these terms.

53. B: User access is handled by an IT professional. More often than not, this person is the database administrator. User access is granted based on the role of the employee. If additional access is found to be needed, managers may submit a request for additional access at the review and approval of the database administrator.

54. D: Medicare conditions of participation: confidentiality of patient records consists of two parts:

- Patient right to confidentiality
- Patient right to access their records in a reasonable time frame.

These same components are illustrated within the HIPAA Privacy Rule, hence the consistent message.

55. C: Disclosing health information involves information that was originated by that facility. Redisclosure is the process of disclosing information that originated by a different provider. Because of this difference, disclosures and redisclosures are governed by different federal and state guidelines.

56. B: If a state has an established retention rate, this shall be upheld as the measure of standard. It is only in scenarios in which a retention rate is not present that the statute of limitations would take effect. Retention rate and statute of limitations are not synonymous terms, nor does the statute of limitations supersede established retention rates.

57. A: Physical safeguards are those that protect buildings and equipment from natural disasters and unauthorized intrusion.

58. C: Destruction certificates are considered best practices in these instances. It is important to note that this documentation should be permanently kept and should never be discarded for any reason.

59. C: PHI should only be sent over a secured medium. PHI should be sent by following the minimum necessary rule, and the communication should only contain the PHI necessary for the participant to complete the task at hand.

60. D: The fact that the system is sending an entire record when there may be a possibility that only part of the record was requested is a violation of the minimum necessary rule in respect to the review of PHI.

61. D: It is vital to contact the facility in which information has been incorrectly sent and verify what has happened with the documentation since its receipt. This is key, especially in cases in which the action is considered to be a breach; notation within the HHS site database is required.

62. A: Although answers B and D are also possible steps to fixing the issue, the best way to do so is through risk management and analysis. Corrective action plans would include interviews with staff, any training, and additional monitoring needed to mitigate risk.

63. D: The governing body over reported breaches would be HHS. Due to the fact that the breach involved fewer than 500 individuals, the media would not require notification.

64. D: Once a patient leaves the premises with PHI that does not belong to them, the scenario goes from incident to breach status. There is no way to quantify how many individuals outside of the patient have reviewed the PHI. Although the patient agreed to discard/shred the documentation, which is important for reporting to HHS, this does not alter the fact that this scenario is a breach.

65. C: When an employee has a family member that is a patient of the facility, access to that patient's records should follow the process for all other patients of the facility with respect to requesting medical records regardless of the patient's age.

66. A: According to regulation, these records should be held for a minimum of 6 years. This 6-year requirement starts from the last effective date of the policy, meaning that any updates should be accounted for and retention dates should be updated to reflect this. Any policies that are kept based on the date of creation when known updates have taken place are not in compliance.

67. C: The patient's gender, birth month, and birth day are considered de-identifiable. However, five-digit ZIP Codes are not considered de-identifiable, especially when used with gender, birth month, and birth day. For example, a ZIP Code associated with a small town, along with the patient's gender and birth information may easily identify a patient.

68. B: BAAs were created out of HIPAA to provide contacts between a covered entity and a vendor with the protection of the PHI at the forefront.

69. A: When a threat to a person or group is identified when reporting to the police, this is covered per the regulatory guidelines within the HIPAA Privacy Rule.

70. C: Breaking the glass is an important feature that allows those who need periodic access to records for a specific reason to do so without having access granted permanently. The feature also allows for an audit trail and a review of the response provided as to why access is needed.

71. C: This is mandated by HHS.

72. D: HIPAA guidelines explain the use of patient identifiers including name and date of birth to identify patients in common areas. Important factors here are that the guidelines outlined certain instances in which this is appropriate and that the payment for services falls within the acceptable purview.

73. A: As a minor patient, the legal guardian(s) of the patient are able to receive information on the patient's behalf. Once that patient turns 18, those rights of the legal guardian are no longer applicable because the patient is deemed to be an adult and is legally able to make their own decisions regarding their care, who is allowed to be contacted/informed of their care, and so forth.

74. C: HIPAA guidelines are specific with regard to fundraising activities. In this scenario, the use of patient demographic data, health insurance status, and dates of service without patient authorization is in compliance because the fundraising partner has a BAA agreement with the hospital.

75. B: It is imperative that any device that contained PHI at any point is reviewed and wiped by the IT department to ensure the protection of that data. The IT department may also properly discard of the device if necessary.

76. D: "Reasonable" is left to the interpretation of each facility, but it must be logically proven if requested within a court of law.

77. D: Patients have a right to refuse to sign an NPP or any other documentation, as stated by HHS.

78. B: Accounting services fall under the category for needed BAAs due to the nature of those services. The HIPAA Privacy Rule outlines those services in which a BAA is required.

79. A: There are guidelines that outline the contents of a patient's legal health record. Among those listed, statistical reports, incident reports, and quality indicators are not included in that list. Their inclusion could pose an issue with regard to the minimum necessary rule.

80. D: PHI may be disposed by a third party as long there is a BAA in place. Currently, there are no requirements stating that only a certain number of records containing PHI may be disposed of by a third party.

81. D: Patient authorizations supersede the minimum-necessary rule.

82. A: HHS is the governing body over the HIPAA Security Rule. The rule contains regulations for the electronic and cybersecurity sectors; it also includes administrative, technical, and physical safeguards.

83. B: Duplicate records are handled by HIM personnel. It is here that the records would be combined, and the duplicate record would be deleted.

84. C: The Institutional Review Board is the governing body over all human research study participants that protects their rights.

85. A: The SELECT function explains what data to retrieve. FROM explains where to get the data, and WHERE serves as a filtering category.

86. C: Data dictionaries serve as a blueprint for the formatting of data. Any changes from what was originally set within the dictionary will need to be updated in the dictionary for accuracy and consistency.

87. C: Scope and critical pathways are not a part of SDLC.

88. B: Utilization management teams are used to review the appropriateness of services provided to patients and the associated costs. This review uses medical necessity, policies, and historical data for parameters when reviewing a case.

89. A: Sentinel events are unforeseen events within the healthcare setting that lead to death or injury (physical or psychological). These events are closely monitored by the Joint Commission as well as hospital administration because many of these events are preventable.

90. A: To calculate the range, the formula is the highest number – the lowest number. This is illustrated in answer choice A.

91. D: Interoperability is a goal of health informatics that impacts the continuity of care for patients by allowing systems to be able to communicate and work with each other in different organizations, demographic areas, and settings.

92. C: Patient portals allow for results, PHI, and other data to be transmitted back and forth from patient to provider through secure means. Text messaging and personal email do not allow for transmission of data securely. PHRs are for the patient to update and track their own health; however, these do not interface with the provider's systems, and therefore the transmission of data is limited or often nonexistent.

93. C: Saving information to the hard drive and sending PHI to personal email addresses are both threats to data security. The use of telemedicine, although using technology, does not provide any form of data security or protection.

94. C: Bus topology involves a single cable connecting all networks together, thus creating a continual line of communication. Hexagonal and train are not types of topology and therefore would not be possible answers for this question.

95. B: IT tickets are methods to document errors or problems that need to be fixed with the system. Statistics and monitoring are ways to document how things are working from a reporting and workflow process review. However, none of the above options capture the feedback of end users other than the use of questionnaires.

96. A: Predictive modeling involves using statistics to predict scenarios. CMS will often use historical data including reports and previous audits to determine what they will review within current prepayment audits.

97. B: Complete use of EHR systems by all communicating facilities provides a means for data to be transmitted and received efficiently and to affect the continuity of care for patients, which are key components of interoperability.

98. B: Physical safeguards support any storage of PHI and/or the equipment containing PHI and the access around those storage areas.

99. B: The NPP outlines a patient's rights in respect to privacy, but it also outlines a facility's due diligence with the patient's information and how the facility intends on using the patient's PHI for services rendered.

100. B: Interoperability between health systems means that information can be shared between facilities. However, to effectively do so, there must be consistency in the standards that are used to govern the activity. Having comprehensive and complete public standards aids in addressing this issue.

101. D: Linear regression would show the strength of a relationship between two variables. It can also be used to determine the dependency of one variable on another.

102. A: For the purposes of data tracking, the department's data flow diagram would need to be updated because the system has changed this process. This is pertinent information to document with any new system or system change/update.

103. C: It is a Joint Commission rule that delinquent records cannot exceed 50% of the average number of discharges.

104. A: Algorithms are a mathematical tool used to determine patterns and trends for the future based on previous data/outcomes and their respective probabilities.

105. B: SDLC includes the installation, configuration, writing, and testing of code. Within SDLC, the develop phase consist of the installation and configuration components. All other components fall in other phases of SDLC.

106. A: Data recovery is a vital part in a business's contingency plan. These plans are developed to serve as a blueprint to lay out how the business will function manually until function is restored. Once restored, data recovery must occur.

107. B: Terminal-digit ordering calls for numbers to be ordered from least to greatest based on the last two digits. This is only done correctly in answer choice B.

108. A: Random sampling is the best-known way of eliminating bias from a sample and is used as a standard of practice during many audits conducted by many entities including CMS.

109. C: Studies have shown that patients who access their own PHRs typically have better health outcomes.

110. D: Telehealth is becoming a popular topic because providers can now provide greater outreach to their patients. Now that coding and reimbursement are being established for this service, HIM professionals should see this service being performed more often.

111. D: Pie charts are best used to show components of a single topic or item.

112. A: Having this in place allows for the facility to have issues documented in an organized way, allows individuals in charge of working the issues see trends/patterns, and allows for timely review.

113. C: Consumer informatics is focused on information structures, components, and processes to promote consumer participation in their own health. This is done through increased patient health literacy, education, and patient-focused informatics.

114. C: The Digital Imaging and Communication in Medicine (DICOM) standard involves information in relation to the transmittal and retrieval of images to diagnostic workstations. Therefore, a review of this standard would be required to ensure that compliance needs are being met.

115. A: Cardinality describes the number of instances in which two or more entities are associated within an entity relationship diagram. This can be a one-to-one, one-to-many, or many-to-many association depending upon the characteristics of the two entities.

116. B: The phased rollout approach consists of rolling out new services in different time frames throughout the organization, whereas the big-bang approach rolls out new services/products all at once throughout the entire facility.

117. C: The Joint Commission monitors hospital delinquency rates. Delinquency rates are very impactful because they can determine whether or not a facility loses accreditation through the Joint Commission.

118. D: All orders should be documented within the EHR. Verbal orders do stand or suffice as in the case of audit, whereas verbal orders cannot be proved. It is important to ensure that all members of the department, EHR team, and HIM team are present to go over how to improve, implement, and monitor going forward.

119. A: This is the best depiction to display and review two or more attributes and their relationship.

120. C: The gross death rate is computed by the total number of reported deaths divided by the total number of discharges. In this case, this would be 15 deaths ÷ 1,000 discharges = 0.015 × 100 = 1.5%.

121. A: Bar coding allows for the proper identification of the right medication to the right patient, but it also ensures the process of transmitting data to the correct record within the EHR.

122. A: Only providing training to the staff or only removing the outdated LCD just tackles part of the problem. Retrospective action is required to ensure that claims accurately report coding and modifiers.

123. C: In order to achieve interoperability with respect to EHRs, the interoperability roadmap suggests consistent standards around the transmission of data nationwide through the aforementioned components listed.

124. A: Every entity should have a data dictionary to fully explain data elements and their meanings. For interoperability, the data elements do not have to be the same, but there have to be data dictionaries in place for facilities to be able to interpret data as intended from one facility to the next.

125. D: The null hypothesis for any experiment is that random chance accounts for the variability in observed results. The alternative hypothesis is what is intending to be demonstrated by the research, i.e., the original hypothesis.

126. C: The types of interoperability are basic, functional, and semantic.

127. C: Structured query language can be high in cost and complex for users, and it only allows for partial database control, which is the opposite of answers A, B, and D.

128. C: Budget negotiations are not a component of determining a vendor's credibility. Credit and reference checks should be done to aid in proving the validity of the vendor and its ability to serve the needs of the facility through services rendered.

129. A: This is shown through the increase of both variables, which in this case illustrates a positive correlation.

130. A: The average is derived by the total LOS days over a given time period. Therefore, the result is all-inclusive, and it provides more accuracy than the range LOS, which only incorporates the extremes or outliers of the data.

131. B: Assumption coding is when a provider or coder selects codes based on the assumption that services were provided but has no actual documentation to support it.

CDI departments can assist by reviewing the documentation and comparing it to what was coded on the claim. They can then render judgments and/or query the physicians and coders about the patient record. Although local code determinations, NCCI edits, and MUE edits can be identified by clinical documentation improvement, these are more so identified at the coding and EHR system level.

132. D: Unbundling involves the reporting of multiple codes to describe a service, when one code accurately reflects the procedure. Upcoding is selecting services and/or diagnoses for the sole purpose of receiving higher reimbursement. Undercoding is conducted when the code billed does not adequately represent the full extent of services provided by a physician or qualified healthcare professional. Multitiered coding is not a term related to HIM.

133. C: The False Claims Act is a federal act that issues sanctions to those who defraud or attempt to defraud the government. The Joint Commission is an accrediting body in health care that requires organizations to follow their standards and regulations. The HITECH Act was made to promote the adoption and meaningful use of health IT.

134. A: Medicare secondary payer (MSP) is a term notifying healthcare facilities that Medicare does not have the primary responsibility for payment pertaining to a patient. An entity relationship model (ERM) is a visual model used to define and show entities and the relationships they possess between other entities. The explanation of benefits (EOB) is the statement sent to beneficiaries of insurance policies to show which costs the insurance has taken care of in relation to their medical services.

135. B: 30-day increments are standard for reporting the aging of accounts.

136. D: Contractual adjustments are those adjustments that are agreed upon through contract negotiations between the facility and insurance companies. The agreements set forth a standard of the percentage of payment that the facility should expect from the insurance company for provided services. Allowance is a term that is mostly used in the revenue cycle realm to describe the amount or threshold of something that is permitted. Revenue recognition involves the period in which revenue is actually considered to be revenue. This term is used mostly in accounting and describes accrual-basis and cash-basis accounting.

137. C: When entities or individuals believe that specific HIPAA violations have been made, they should file a complaint with the HHS through the Office for Civil Rights (OCR) within 180 days of the violation. The OCR is then responsible for investigating the HIPAA complaint and producing a report generated in a letter to the individual(s) affected, with appropriate actions made if necessary. Violations relating to health and safety that occur in hospitals that participate in Medicare/Medicaid programs should be reported to the CMS per the CMS Conditions of Participation (CoP). The Joint Commission recommends that patient safety issues, such as sentinel events, be self-reported so that appropriate root-cause analyses can be performed for future prevention measures. Health care compliance-related violations (such as fraud) should be reported to the HHS via the Office of Inspector General.

138. A: Patients have a right to report any medical identity theft to the HHS Office of Civil Rights.

139. D: Insurance verification is a front-end process that is considered to be one of the first pivotal steps in the revenue cycle process. Charge capture, CDM management, and clinical documentation are all back-end revenue cycle processes that would not include the efforts conducted at registration.

140. C: In an effort to stay abreast of compliance changes within health care, it is necessary to check OIG work plans, ICD-10 CM and ICD-PCS guidelines, and changes in reimbursement systems. Previous-year updates to ICD-10, CPT, and HCPCS coding systems are no longer relevant because updates to these codes happen annually and therefore should not be referenced for current-year compliance references.

141. B: Medicare serves those individuals who are 65 and older. TRICARE serves active-duty military or other eligible members. Commercial insurance services the vast population often given to individuals through their employers.

142. C: HMOs are prepaid voluntary health plans that provide their members with services in return for premiums paid on a monthly basis. Within this plan, members must visit healthcare providers on the HMO list other than for emergency services.

143. B: Coordination of benefits is a process used to discover and validate which insurance is considered primary and which is considered secondary when a patient presents with more than one insurance provider. This process is key in the reimbursement process and aids in reducing the chances of payment duplication.

144. C: Preauthorization is a requirement that is made by insurance companies to cause the member to get permission prior to receiving the procedure to ensure that the member's insurance will pay for the service.

145. B: LOS days, total days in AR, and days in total discharged, no final bill, are all internal metrics for a healthcare facility. In order to review the diagnosis-related group mix of patients in relation to other hospitals, the hospital would need to use the case-mix index.

146. D: The removal of modifiers from a claim once it is discovered that it is unnecessary to do so will result in a clean claim, and if it is performed correctly should not result in a denial. However, if a service is stated as noncovered by the patient's insurance and has medical necessity and/or preauthorization issues, these all fall under the common reasons for healthcare denials.

147. C: Government payers have the right to exclude individuals found to have been involved with the illegal receipt of payments from the government. This exclusion makes it so that the individual cannot participate in federal programs, meaning that if the person excluded is working for a facility that receives payments from government payers, then that facility would be at risk of losing those contracts.

148. B: Extrapolation is an auditing method that reviews a small subset of claims, finds an error rate, and then applies that error rate over a large subset of claims over a certain period of time. For example, if within an audit of 5 claims an 80% error rate was found, with the extrapolation method the auditor could apply that error rate to 1,000 claims over a 3-year period. This would result in substantial paybacks to the government payer.

149. C: Although compliance, hospital billing, and charge data master teams are all involved in the process and are ultimately affected by the education provided, it is the duty of CDI and the HIM teams to ensure the training/education needed is provided.

150. C: Claim scrubbers are set up to provide an internal auditing system to ensure that the claim passes certain logic and edits prior to being submitted to the payer. If a claim is sent to the claim scrubber and fails, this will often result in it being sent to work queues to be manually worked on by human staff to address issues with the claim.

151. D: Accounts receivable days start once the claim has been billed to the payer.

152. A: Medicare serves those individuals who are 65 and older. Medicaid serves those members who are of low income. Commercial insurance serves the vast majority of the population often being given to individuals through their employers.

153. C: Value-based care is the methodology in which payment should be remitted to providers and healthcare facilities based on the quality of care provided to the patient. This level of quality is determined by measures established by CMS, and results are compared nationally to other healthcare facilities in the same lines of business. Value-based care is being pushed more to the forefront as health care moves away from fee for service.

154. D: Submitting a claim to an insurance company from a healthcare facility is the standard way to request payment within the healthcare system.

155. A: Avoidable denials are those denials that can be resolved by changes within the facility. This could be done through improvements within workflows, education to the staff and or providers, etc. Authorization and registration denials can be altered based on changes made by the facility and are therefore deemed avoidable.

156. C: A patient's discharge and/or admission date is not included in the calculation of days in accounts receivable.

157. D: Key performance indicators allow for healthcare organizations to benchmark and trend data to identity weaknesses and measures of success.

158. A: A mission statement spells out an organization's purpose in the specific industry that they are conducting business in. A strategic plan is created by top-level management to set the priorities of the organizations based on an analysis of the organization's strengths and weaknesses. SMART goals — which stands for specific, measurable, achievable, realistic, and time-bound — are a model for achieving optimal goal results.

159. D: Emotional intelligence defines an individual's ability to view and analyze their own behavior based on the behavioral responses of others, including self-awareness, self-regulation, motivation, empathy, and social skills.

160. C: The early majority includes those who think through the accepting process of new ideas and are the liaisons between the early and late adopters. Early adopters often are considered local opinion leaders. These individuals are more than likely the leaders within the organization.

161. B: A vision statement is a description of an organization's future goals and optimal results. A strategic plan is created by top-level management to set the priorities of the organization based on an analysis of the organization's strength and weaknesses. SMART goals are a model for achieving optimal goal results.

162. A: Gantt charts show dependent relationships between activities and current established schedules.

163. C: Autonomy represents patients' rights to choose their own course of treatment and/or care. This includes the right to refuse treatment. Beneficence is aiding in providing services that benefit others. Altruism is the standard that the whole is greater than the sum of its parts. Egoism is only considering oneself in the decision-making process/activities.

164. B: Although equality and communication are important within HIM, these elements are not stand-alone categories with respect to the AHIMA Code of Ethics.

165. A: The AHIMA code of ethics serves seven purposes.

166. D: Although the more direct ethical obligations of HIM professionals are to the patient as well as the healthcare sector, there is also an obligation to the public to improve health outcomes.

167. B: Complete job descriptions include the qualifications needed to perform the job and will also include the synopsis of the position requirements. Although some jobs may post salary ranges, ways to contact the hiring manager, and/or discuss promotional growth, this is not a requirement, and it is up to the employer's discretion as to whether or not this is made public.

168. A: Job specifications contain the required educational level, skills and abilities, experience, etc. The job description outlines the work that will be performed by the employee. Job specifications are included within job descriptions.

169. B: Control within conflict management involves a manager setting ground rules to structure interactions. Constructive confrontation includes parties meeting with a third party to produce a mutual understanding. Within HIM, mediation is considered a part of grievance management and not conflict management.

170. B: Coaching goes beyond teaching. Coaching often includes counseling, serving as a problem solver, as well as being a resource person.

171. A: Mentoring, in most cases, is done through a one-to-one pairing of mentor and mentee. This differs from coaching in that coaching may consist of a coach that guides a group of individuals for a given purpose.

172. D: The attainable standard involves having a reasonable standard that individuals can actually achieve. The equitable standard involves accountability. The significant standard describes the importance in meeting the standard, but also that the effort put forth to meet the standard is worth it.

173. B: The current ratio is the only answer choice applicable to liquidity. It represents the organization's ability to pay current liabilities and current assets.

174. C: Since Evan is creating a control to find a pre-existing error, this would be categorized as a detective control. Preventive controls seek to prevent errors before they occur. Corrective control takes place once an error has been detected, the controls are put in place to correct the issue, and it is ensured that is it not reoccurring.

175. A: It is important to remember that in this example we are discussing expenses and revenue. With regard to expenses, an actual amount greater than the budgeted amount is considered unfavorable. However, in respect to revenue, an actual amount greater than the budgeted amount is considered favorable.

176. C: Cost–benefit analysis is a review of whether the cost of an item, opportunity, etc. outweighs the benefit. In this example, the cost of keeping the current machine outweighed the benefit once it was discovered that it would be cheaper to buy a new machine with a warranty.

177. A: The opportunity cost is the potential loss of benefit from other options when one option is selected. The profit period is not a term associated with this curriculum. The rate of return is a gain or loss of an investment over a period of time.

178. C: Utilitarianism is the concept of making decisions/choices that provide the greatest benefit to the most people. Beneficence involves promoting the good of others or providing services that benefit others. The least-harm concept encompasses situations that have two less-than-ideal options, but one is selected based on the fact that it would provide less harm than the other. Deontology is guided decision making based on action and not on results.

179. B: Blanket authorizations give the ROI professional permission to release any and all information going forward from the date of signature. Release of information is the concept behind releasing information at the patient's request and the rights associated with that from the patient's and the facility's perspective. Authorization review is not an HIM concept.

180. D: Competitor analysis is an external assessment in which data on the organization's competitors are collected and analyzed to compare, benchmark, and trend the comparisons between the organization and others within the same industry. All of the other answer choices involve internal assessments.

RHIA Practice Test #2

1. What does the process of system configuration consist of?
   a. Prepping the system or software application to meet the needs of the specific organization in which it will be implemented
   b. Setting access controls so only authorized users are permitted to retrieve data
   c. Downloading only the most up-to-date applications
   d. Running antivirus scans to detect and remove malicious software

2. A famous celebrity was recently admitted to your hospital for emergency surgery. It has been recommended that during this patient's stay, audit logs be conducted to determine if inappropriate access to the patient's protected health information (PHI) has occurred. What type of measure is this?
   a. Administrative safeguard
   b. Physical safeguard
   c. Addressable safeguard
   d. Technical safeguard

3. What performance improvement tool would be the best option to identify the potential root causes of problems?
   a. Flowchart
   b. Fishbone diagram
   c. Pareto chart
   d. Check sheet

4. A patient who was recently treated in your facility has paid in full for all services out of pocket (this patient does have insurance). The patient has requested that all information regarding this visit remain private and not be shared with their insurance company. Is this an appropriate request, and should the healthcare facility comply with this patient's request?
   a. Yes, because the patient paid out of pocket (in full), the insurance company has no responsibility for payment.
   b. Yes, a patient can withhold any treatment information from their insurance company at any time.
   c. No, because the insurance company may cover the costs of these services.
   d. No, because this individual has insurance and healthcare services should never be kept from their insurer.

5. What is the time frame for completing an operative report for a high-risk procedure?
   a. Whenever the provider has enough time to dedicate to documentation
   b. No more than 1 week following the procedure
   c. Immediately after a procedure is completed
   d. Within 30 days of the procedure

6. A manager has created an image to help her visualize a defined workspace as well as functions or other related tasks performed in that designated area to determine how they are related. What kind of visualization tool has the manager created?
   a. Work distribution chart
   b. Dashboard
   c. Movement diagram
   d. Heat map

7. Which of the following payment methods reimburses providers using a fixed amount for each of their patients enrolled in a managed care plan?
   a. Fee-for-service
   b. Bundled rate
   c. Capitated rate
   d. Pay for performance

8. A summary of job position requirements, the job's purpose/function, and the qualifications needed to perform the job can all be found in which document?
   a. Job description
   b. Job evaluation
   c. Job ranking
   d. Job classification

9. A 60-year-old female patient was admitted to the hospital complaining of a severe headache. The nurse measuring her vital signs has alerted the provider that the patient has a low blood pressure reading. The provider requested a CT scan and urinalysis (UA). The UA showed a decrease in the glomerular filtration rate, and the CT showed a ruptured brain aneurysm. The patient was taken to emergency surgery for microvascular clipping. What was the chief complaint?
   a. Brain aneurysm
   b. Dehydration
   c. Low blood pressure
   d. Severe headache

10. Which of the following is considered a common model and iterative approach used by course creators and training designers for successful training development?
    a. HITSC
    b. FASB
    c. DIKW
    d. ADDIE

11. Which of the following would NOT be information necessary to define in a data dictionary for data fields or columns?
    a. An entity relationship diagram
    b. The name, type, and length of each data field
    c. Clear definitions of each data field
    d. Allowed values that can be used in each data field

12. Which of the following is considered the most recognizable component of the problem-oriented health record?

   a. Source-oriented record
   b. Integrated format
   c. SOAP format
   d. Legal health record

13. An HIM director is currently determining how long medical records should be kept according to the Medicare Conditions of Participation requirements. A health record created on March 10, 2010, should have been retained until at least which of the following dates?

   a. March 10, 2013
   b. March 10, 2015
   c. March 10, 2016
   d. March 10, 2020

14. A general practitioner recently saw a patient who complained of fatigue and dizziness. The general practitioner requests that the patient get blood work done and decides to send the patient to a clinical laboratory owned by his brother because he has a financial relationship with this entity and will be compensated. What law did this doctor violate?

   a. Right-to-know laws
   b. Good Samaritan laws
   c. The Stark Law
   d. Private law

15. A risk management team is tracking the number of medication errors resolved with the help of clinical decision support in December. The following errors were resolved: Wrong patient (70), wrong dose (30), wrong drug (60), and wrong route (20). What data in this summary report are incorrectly represented?

Resolved Medication Errors

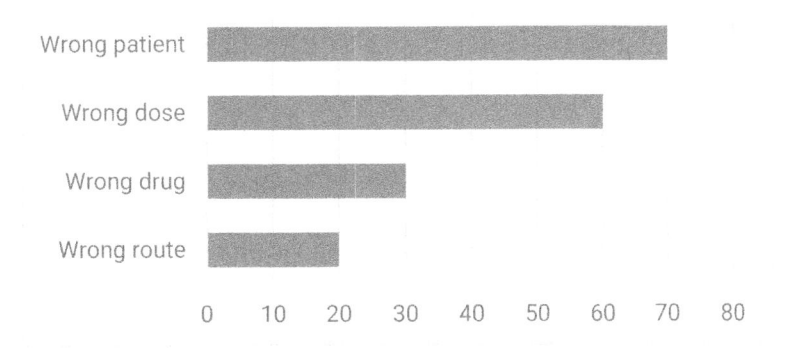

Category	Value
Wrong patient	~70
Wrong dose	~60
Wrong drug	~30
Wrong route	~20

   a. The value for the wrong patient is incorrectly represented.
   b. The values for the wrong drug and wrong dose should be switched.
   c. The title is incorrectly represented.
   d. All elements of the graph are represented correctly.

16. A coding supervisor wants to display the entire coding process from start to finish to highlight relevant variables, such as steps associated with the process and individuals responsible for each step. Which visualization tool would be most appropriate to display this information?
   a. Swimlane diagram
   b. Force-field analysis
   c. Run chart
   d. Affinity grouping

17. A patient has presented to the emergency department in critical condition after being struck by a car while riding his bicycle. After registering the patient, the department discovers that the patient does not have health insurance and would be unable to pay for their treatment. It is suggested to transfer the patient to a hospital 12 miles away to avoid treating a patient without insurance coverage. What section of the Consolidated Omnibus Budget Reconciliation Act (COBRA) obliges a hospital that participates in Medicare to stabilize and treat patients regardless of their insurance status?
   a. NCCI
   b. ERISA
   c. FMLA
   d. EMTALA

18. Six Sigma's DMAIC method used for business transformation consists of five phases including define, measure, analyze, improve, and _____.
   a. calculate
   b. confirm
   c. control
   d. coordinate

19. A hospital recently purchased a computerized provider order entry system for $150,000. The hospital has a liability from a long-term bank loan of $100,000 for this purchase. The revenue generated from this purchase was $36,000. Using this information, calculate the return on investment.
   a. 43%
   b. 67%
   c. 24%
   d. 36%

20. What functionality should be used with caution in the EHR system environment to ensure the continued integrity of health data?
   a. Patient access
   b. Audit trails
   c. Copy and paste
   d. Public database access

21. A patient requested a copy of her medical records on March 3. Her request should be responded to by what date?

   a. March 16
   b. March 24
   c. April 1
   d. April 30

22. A new patient presents to your office for an appointment and provides two healthcare insurance carrier cards (Medicare and Medicaid). What is the most appropriate action to take in this situation?

   a. Create claims for both insurance carriers.
   b. Do not create claims for either insurance carrier.
   c. Determine which insurance carrier is primary and which one is secondary.
   d. Ask the patient which one they would prefer to be billed.

23. A 65-year-old patient presented to the emergency department with meningitis due to African trypanosomiasis. Based on this information, what would be the correct code selection?

   > **B56.0**—Gambiense trypanosomiasis infection due to *Trypanosoma brucei gambiense*
   > West African sleeping sickness
   > **G02**—Meningitis

   a. B56.0
   b. G02
   c. [G02], B56.0
   d. B56.0, [G02]

24. What is the standardized programming language used to communicate with and manage relational databases?

   a. Java
   b. Object-oriented languages
   c. Python
   d. Structured Query Language

25. Important considerations for data governance do NOT include which of the following?

   a. The mapping of data flow
   b. The needs of data consumers
   c. The classification and categorization of data
   d. The application of internal regulations only

26. Which of the following is a process whereby government-associated agencies grant legal authorization for a healthcare professional to practice an occupation?

   a. Credentialization
   b. Accreditation
   c. Licensure
   d. Authorization

27. A quality improvement team performs an internal and external assessment of its organization. It has determined that it has an emerging market and increased access to interns. How would these be classified in a SWOT analysis?
   a. Strength
   b. Weakness
   c. Opportunity
   d. Threat

28. Based on the financial data listed below, what was Gibson's net income?

Gibson Healthcare Financial Data 12/31/202X	
Cash	$350,000
Accounts receivable	$100,000
Building	$2,000,000
Land	$500,000
Accounts payable	$250,000
Mortgage	$900,500
Revenue	$3,500,500
Expenses	$2,000,500

   a. $1,500,000
   b. $350,000
   c. $3,300,000
   d. $450,000

29. Robert is the custodian of health records at his medical practice and has been called on to appear for a legal proceeding of a malpractice suit. What role is Robert responsible for regarding the medical documentation presented in the case?
   a. Determine if the provider authenticated the record
   b. Determine if the principal diagnosis of a patient was accurately assigned.
   c. Testify that medical care was appropriately documented.
   d. Testify to the admissibility of the record.

30. An HIM manager wants to resolve an issue between two employees using a specific conflict management solution. The manager has decided to let one of the employees have their way because the other employee does not care as strongly about the issue of concern. What is the conflict management style used in this scenario?
   a. Compromising
   b. Avoiding
   c. Collaborating
   d. Accommodating

31. Who has the responsibility of guaranteeing healthcare record documentation quality?
   a. Provider
   b. Data steward
   c. Health information professional
   d. Quality manager

32. A CDI specialist has begun reviewing documentation from patient's records weeks or even months after patients have been discharged to gather data for decisions and to identify trends. What type of chart review is the CDI specialist performing?

   a. Prospective review
   b. Medical necessity review
   c. Retrospective review
   d. Complex review

33. Code the following scenario: A patient underwent posterior arthrodesis of 7 vertebral segments with a cast.

> **22800**—Arthrodesis, posterior, for spinal deformity, with or without cast; up to 6 vertebral segments
> **22802**—Arthrodesis, posterior, for spinal deformity, with or without cast; 7–12 vertebral segments
> **22808**—Arthrodesis, anterior, for spinal deformity, with or without cast; 2–3 vertebral segments
> **22810**—Arthrodesis, anterior, for spinal deformity, with or without cast; 4–7 vertebral segments

   a. 22800, 22802
   b. 22802
   c. 22810
   d. 22808, 22810

34. Who has the legal right to obtain the medical records of another person without requiring a signed authorization ROI form?

> 1. The nurse of a past patient
> 2. The parent of an emancipated minor
> 3. The caretaker of an incompetent adult
> 4. The spouse of a patient
> 5. The guardian of a 12-year-old minor

   a. 3 and 5
   b. 1 and 2
   c. 4 and 5
   d. 1 and 3

35. Which of the following is NOT a component of a records retention program?

   a. Determine the location and format of record storage.
   b. Conduct an inventory of the facility's records.
   c. Destroy records when they are close to the end of the retention period.
   d. Assign each record a specific time for preservation.

36. A hospital is trying to alleviate staffing shortages by creating floating positions. Workers in these positions learn to perform the jobs of several employees so they can provide help wherever assistance is needed. What kind of training is best suited to accomplish this objective?
   a. Mentoring
   b. Cross-training
   c. Compliance training
   d. Outsourcing

37. Trevor has been tracking patients' recent lengths of stay to see if there are any trends. Trevor decides to present his summary report to the admissions department and uses the mean length of stay as a facility statistic. After examining the table below, what would be the biggest problem with using this measure of central tendency?

Patient	Length of Stay
A	3
B	7
C	4
D	6
E	28
F	5
G	3

   a. The mean can be sensitive to extreme values falling outside the normal range and can distort the portrayal of the data set's measure of central tendency.
   b. There is no problem; Trevor used the appropriate measure of central tendency based on the information provided.
   c. It would be mathematically incorrect to use the mean length of stay.
   d. Using the mode of the data set would be the most accurate representation of the length of stay's measure of central tendency.

38. The image below is an example of what kind of data analysis tool?

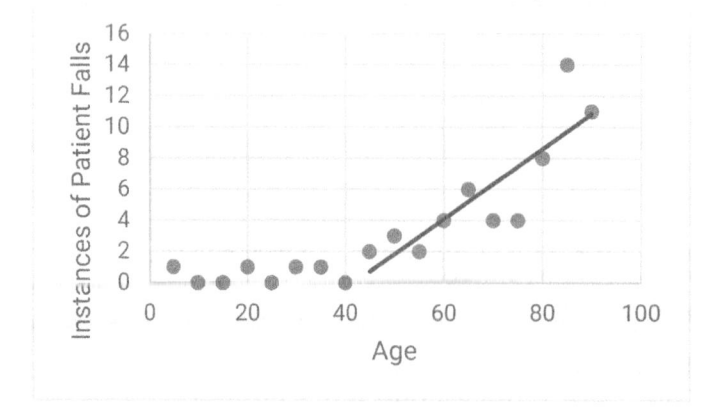

   a. Radar chart
   b. Line graph
   c. Histogram
   d. Scatterplot

39. The performance improvement team is examining a summary report based on employee turnover trends over the past 4 years. What action should the team take based on the data displayed in the graph below?

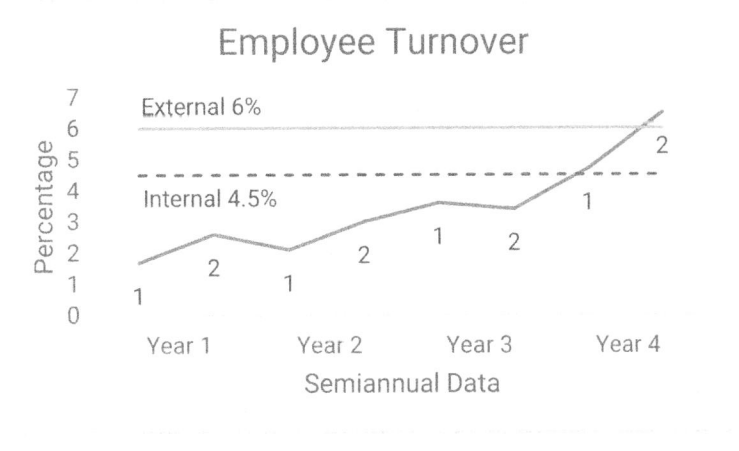

Employee Turnover

a. Examine the cause for the low employee turnover rate in year 1.
b. Take no action because employee satisfaction has steadily increased over the past 4 years.
c. Take no action because employee turnover rates cannot be influenced.
d. Examine the cause for the high employee turnover rate in year 4.

40. The HIM director has asked you to create a productivity report based on the results from the last audit. According to the director, the HIM department is scanning 300 pages and filing 174 pages per hour. The department is meeting the productivity standards for scanning. However, they are only meeting 50% of the filing standard. How many more pages per hour must the department file to meet the filing productivity standard?

a. 261 pages
b. 174 pages
c. 87 pages
d. 126 pages

41. What Latin term describes decisions made on landmark cases that set a precedence that lower courts in the same jurisdiction are expected to follow regarding similar legal cases?

a. *Respondeat superior*
b. *Stare decisis*
c. *Res ipsa loquitur*
d. *Subpoena ad testificandum*

42. For a contract to be considered valid and legally enforceable, it must contain all of the following EXCEPT:

a. Contractual offer
b. Contract acceptance
c. Contractual consideration
d. Contract payment

43. Of the options listed, which of the following would NOT be considered malware?
    a. Rootkits
    b. Bugs
    c. Keyloggers
    d. Trojans

44. During a recent follow-up appointment, a patient discusses their medical condition with their provider. What is the legal term that best represents this type of communication occurring between the patient and their physician?
    a. Clinical communication
    b. Private communication
    c. Privileged communication
    d. Open communication

45. Project management is used to help control activities when undertaking significant organizational changes. When implementing project management, all of the following are considered core constraints EXCEPT:
    a. Budget
    b. Belief
    c. Scope
    d. Schedule

46. Healthcare facilities collect, process, and store various data to help support organizational operations. This information can identify patients, providers, and the location of encounters, among other things. What kind of data is this information considered?
    a. Administrative data
    b. Operational data
    c. Clinical data
    d. Financial data

47. A provider performed a sigmoidoscopy with the removal of polyps. The clinical documentation does not specify whether hot biopsy forceps, the snare technique, or the ablation method was used to remove the polyps. Based on this information, what would be the most appropriate action to take regarding code selection?
    a. Select the code of the most common polyp removal method.
    b. Query the physician regarding the method that was used in this encounter.
    c. Select the code that would result in the highest reimbursement.
    d. The removal technique does not matter, and the selection of any polyp removal code will have the same impact.

48. A patient has requested copies of their medical records and was informed by the ROI specialist that there will be charges associated with this ROI request. Is the statement that the ROI specialist has relayed to the patient true? Why or why not?
    a. No, patients should never be charged for copies of their own PHI.
    b. Yes, cost-based fees can be charged for copying the PHI.
    c. No, charges for PHI can only occur when someone else makes the request.
    d. Yes, patients are always charged for receiving copies of their PHI.

49. Which of the following is an itemized list with details of services provided to a patient that is sent to a patient's healthcare insurance company to calculate reimbursement?
    a. Remittance advice
    b. Chargemaster
    c. Superbill
    d. Advanced beneficiary notice

50. Accession number 04-0056 has been assigned to a patient in a cancer registry. What do the first two digits of this accession number represent?
    a. The year a patient was first seen
    b. The type of cancer a patient is diagnosed with
    c. The patient's stage of cancer
    d. The facility's unique ID number

51. Over the past 6 months, a hospital's pediatric floor has reported 45 new cases of respiratory syncytial virus. These 45 cases represent 25% of this hospital's pediatric population. This rate represents the:
    a. Prevalence
    b. Frequency
    c. Incidence
    d. Density

52. Which healthcare professionals must determine whether an individual or entity can rightfully access PHI?
    a. HIM professionals
    b. Attending physicians
    c. IT professionals
    d. Healthcare administrators

53. What program was developed by CMS to promote accurate coding and prevent improper reporting of incorrect code combinations?
    a. NCHS
    b. HIPAA
    c. AAMT
    d. NCCI

54. An established patient arrives at a doctor's office for their visit. During the check-in process, the patient provides the receptionist with her driving license. The receptionist notices that it is different than what is on file. The patient has the same name, but her date of birth and address have changed. The patient also looks quite different from the photo on her ID. The receptionist ignores these inconsistencies and sends the patient to see the physician. Later, it was discovered that this individual had committed medical identity theft. A detailed training on which fraud statute should occur to prevent situations like this from happening again?
    a. Red Flag Rule
    b. Healthcare Fraud Statute
    c. Exclusion Provisions
    d. False Claims Act

55. After implementing a new EHR system, the performance improvement team notices that many physicians are reluctant to use the system. The majority claim they are frustrated, stating that it is challenging to navigate the interface and that it seems too time-consuming to explore its functionalities. The performance improvement team was not prepared for these project dependencies. Of the options listed, what is the most appropriate course of action to address the physician's concerns?
   a. Install a system that the providers feel more comfortable using.
   b. Allow the physicians to figure out the EHR system at their own pace.
   c. Provide support staff and implement training programs for the physicians.
   d. Have super users perform the physician's data entry and actions in the EHR system.

56. A covered entity has released information requested by a patient's insurance company after ensuring that an authorization form for the ROI was signed by the patient. Later that day, the patient presented to the HIM department to revoke the authorization for the ROI. What actions will result from the information being released earlier that day?
   a. The covered entity would have to pay a fine for committing a breach violation.
   b. The covered entity would be placed on probation and lose access rights for 6 months.
   c. The covered entity would be protected under the Privacy Rule.
   d. The covered entity would face legal percussions.

57. When an individual suspects being a victim of medical identity theft, which agency should the person file a complaint with?
   a. Office of Civil Rights (OCR)
   b. Centers for Disease Control and Prevention (CDC)
   c. Federal Trade Commission (FTC)
   d. Centers for Medicare and Medicaid Services (CMS)

58. William Jones has presented to a physician's office requesting medical records on behalf of his wife, Bethany. He tells the ROI specialist that his wife is at home sick with the flu and she has sent him to receive a copy of her medical records. How should the ROI specialist proceed in this situation?
   a. Release a copy of the medical records to Mr. Jones.
   b. Request that Mr. Jones sign an authorization for the ROI form before releasing any records.
   c. Inform Mr. Jones that his wife will have to sign an authorization for the ROI form, and she must specify that her husband can receive her medical records.
   d. Allow Mr. Jones to view a copy of his wife's medical record, but deny him from taking the copy home.

59. Which part of the revenue management life cycle includes clinical documentation, charge capture, case management, and coding?
   a. Front end
   b. Middle process
   c. Back end
   d. Closing end

60. Given the information provided below, what would the case-mix index be?

MS-DRG	MDC	Type	MS-DRG Title	Weight	Discharges	Geometric Mean	Arithmetic Mean
143	03	MED	Other ear, nose, mouth, and throat OR procedures with MCC	1.2468	20	4.2	4.5
144	03	MED	Other ear, nose, mouth, and throat OR procedures with CC	0.6527	20	3.4	3.9
145	03	MED	Other ear, nose, mouth, and throat OR procedures w/o CC/MCC	0.9362	10	2.7	3.1

a. 0.94704
b. 3.58
c. 3.98
d. 0.57238

61. What is considered to be the best approach to training staff members on EHR applications?

a. Only offer in-house training so employees can ask questions as they arise.
b. Offer online training so employees can learn the content at their own pace.
c. Implement a variety of training methods to accommodate various learning styles.
d. Create training videos that employees can watch at any time.

62. The admissions department has implemented a new patient registration system to mitigate an increase in registration errors. A few months after the new system was first implemented, similar errors continued occurring. Based on these facts, what is the most likely cause of this issue?

a. The old system was infected by malware.
b. There were underlying human registration processes that were not addressed and corrected first.
c. The new system had not been properly installed.
d. Both patient registration systems had the same defects.

63. During the e-discovery process, the director of HIM at your facility has advised that the patient records involved with the litigation be specially tracked and handled to avoid any alteration or destruction of these documents. What is the most appropriate term used to describe the HIM director's request?

a. Preservation of evidence
b. Spoliation
c. Legal hold
d. Disposition

64. Many medical claims submitted by one coding specialist have been denied due to incorrect code assignments. The coding compliance officer decides to review a random sample of 50 cases coded by the specialist over the past month. What kind of audit is the compliance officer conducting?
   a. Random audit
   b. External audit
   c. IRS audit
   d. Focused audit

65. A patient was recently admitted to a hospital and has elected to opt out of the facility directory. What would be the most appropriate action to take in this situation?
   a. Inform the patient that they cannot opt out of the facility directory.
   b. Ask the patient why they want to opt out of the facility directory before removing them.
   c. Assure the patient that only family members will be provided information about their health.
   d. Have the patient sign an opt-out form before removing them.

66. What character and symbol recognition technology has the potential of reducing medication errors?
   a. Computerized provider order entry
   b. Scanning
   c. Barcoding
   d. Vector graphic data

67. What type of analysis is conducted to determine how vital the information in health information systems is with regard to day-to-day operations and patient care?
   a. Classification analysis
   b. Perspective analysis
   c. Requirements analysis
   d. Criticality analysis

68. Which of the following systems allows patient access to all or a portion of their health records that are maintained by their physician?
   a. EHR
   b. Patient portal
   c. Clinical web portal
   d. Personal health record

69. One way to prepare and support end users in EHR applications is to determine if they have any prior experience using these systems and to assess any experiences they have had or opinions they hold on the organization's systems. What data collection method would be the most appropriate to use to obtain this information?
   a. Sampling methods
   b. Interviews
   c. Observations
   d. Questionnaire surveys

70. As part of the EMPI's ongoing maintenance program, the MPI coordinator must resolve duplicates, overlays, and overlap errors found within the EMPI. What is the term used to describe this maintenance process?

a. Identification
b. Cleanup
c. Reduction
d. Declutter

71. The legal doctrine established by the landmark case *Tarasoff v. Regents of the University of California* of 1976 resulted in the Tarasoff Rule. What legal health concept does this rule enforce?

a. Duty to warn
b. Corporate negligence
c. Need for advance directives
d. Implicit right to privacy

72. Johnathan is an HIM analyst who is inspecting the medical record of Jane Smith while she is still a patient in the facility to ensure that all entries are complete and authenticated. What is this process called?

a. Quantitative analysis
b. Predictive analysis
c. Concurrent review
d. Retrospective review

73. The following graph was created by tracking the number of productive hours logged by the facility's coding department. What change could be made to make this visualization of the productivity report more effective?

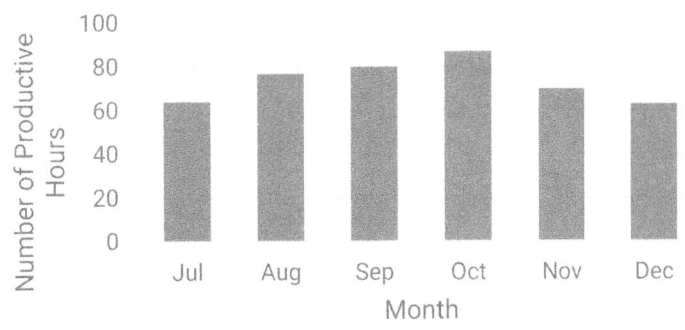

a. Use a different title to describe the graph.
b. Present the data as a line plot.
c. Present the data as a pie chart.
d. Increase the number of productive hours per month.

74. What clinical terminology is used to facilitate a universal method of reporting laboratory observations?
   a. LOINC
   b. CPT
   c. SNOMED CT
   d. RxNorm

75. A healthcare organization wants to solicit a small group of prescreened potential EHR vendors. A structured document is used to compare the functionality and feasibility of each system so the organization can make an informed decision on which bid best fits its requirements. Which of the following best describes this process?
   a. Request for proposal
   b. Request for information
   c. Request for quotation
   d. Request for services

76. Given the following table, which facility would be considered to have a tier 3 violation according to the HIPAA Omnibus Rule?

		Data Breach	
Facility	Affected Individuals	Violation Category	Action Taken
1	45	Willful neglect	Corrected within 30 days
2	56	Lack of knowledge	N/A
3	507	Reasonable cause	Corrected within 30 days
4	282	Willful neglect	Not corrected within 30 days

   a. Facility 1
   b. Facility 2
   c. Facility 3
   d. Facility 4

77. What is the term used to describe the process of furnishing proof of authorship of medical record documentation?
   a. Standardization
   b. Identification
   c. Authorization
   d. Authentication

78. During an accreditation survey, a technique was used to assess operational systems and processes by closely examining the experiences of selected patients. Which of the following approaches best describes this procedure?
   a. Tracer methodology
   b. Audit trail
   c. Content analysis
   d. Historical research

79. Covered entities must notify the secretary of the Department of Health and Human Services (HHS) on PHI breaches that affect up to 500 individuals no later than which of the following?
    a. 30 days after the breach was discovered
    b. 60 days after the end of the calendar year in which the breach was discovered
    c. 1 year after the breach was discovered
    d. 3 years after the end of the calendar year in which the breach was discovered

80. Which of the following standards is implemented to avoid confusion and variations in the naming of medical procedures and conditions?
    a. Transaction standards
    b. Privacy standards
    c. Data structure and content standards
    d. Vocabulary standards

81. All of the following would typically be included in an HIM department's operational budget EXCEPT:
    a. Computers
    b. Benefits
    c. Payroll
    d. Office supplies

82. A patient had undergone a cryoablation of a skin lesion on her right breast. Which of the following is the correct ICD-10-PCS code for this procedure?

Section	Body System	Root Operation	Body Part	Approach	Device	Qualifier
Medical and surgical 0	Skin and breast H	Destruction 5	Right breast T	External X	No device Z	No qualifier Z

Section	Body System	Root Operation	Body Part	Approach	Device	Qualifier
Medical and surgical 0	Skin and breast H	Drainage 9	Right breast T	External X	Drainage device 0	No qualifier Z

Section	Body System	Root Operation	Body Part	Approach	Device	Qualifier
Medical and surgical 0	Skin and breast H	Excision B	Right breast T	Percutaneous 3	No device Z	Diagnostic X

Section	Body System	Root Operation	Body Part	Approach	Device	Qualifier
Medical and surgical 0	Skin and breast H	Extirpation C	Right breast T	External X	No device Z	No qualifier Z

   a. 0H5TXZZ
   b. 0H9TX0Z
   c. 0HBT3ZX
   d. 0HCTXZZ

83. A new patient arrives at a doctor's office for his first appointment. He is provided a notice explaining how and when his PHI can be used or disclosed. This patient has been asked to sign a form stating that he has received the notice. What type of document was this patient provided?
   a. Notice of privacy practices
   b. Advance Beneficiary Notice of Noncoverage form
   c. Business associate agreement
   d. Medicare summary notice

84. A patient was recently discharged from a psychiatric unit at a local hospital. A few weeks later, the patient called the medical records department to request access to the psychotherapy notes created during their stay. What is the appropriate way to respond to this patient's request?
   a. Inform the patient that psychotherapy notes are not released to patients.
   b. The release of psychotherapy notes to a patient must be approved by a licensed healthcare professional.
   c. Deny the request because it is too soon following the patient's discharge date.
   d. Allow the request only after an authorization ROI form is signed by the patient.

85. An HIM professional has received an ROI request from a patient's employer. The employer is seeking medical records about a patient's recent work-related injury. From the options listed here, what would be the most appropriate action for the HIM professional to take?
   a. Contact the workers' compensation specialist and ask for advice.
   b. Release the minimum necessary PHI to the employer for workers' compensation purposes.
   c. Require the employer to sign an authorization form first.
   d. Inform the employer that written authorization from the patient will be required first.

86. All of the following statistical techniques can be used to determine the probability of claims being fraudulent EXCEPT:
   a. Decision trees
   b. Flowcharts
   c. Logistic regressions
   d. Cluster analyses

87. What portion of a medical record is displayed below?

> **Constitutional:** Weight loss, no fever, no fatigue
> **Eyes:** No changes in vision, no eye pain
> **ENT:** No sinus pressure, no tooth pain, no hearing loss
> **Respiratory:** Cough, no wheezing or sputum production
> **Skin:** No rash, no changes in skin lesions

   a. Family history
   b. Present illness
   c. Review of systems
   d. Diagnosis

88. A coder noticed conflicting information while reviewing a patient's medical record. The coder used the organization's routine method of obtaining clarification by consulting the physician who originated the document. What kind of communication tool has the coder used to clarify the documentation?

   a. Investigation
   b. Physician interview
   c. Inspection
   d. Physician query

89. Unlike the traditional fee-for-service reimbursement method, in which providers are paid for each service that they perform, what do value-based purchasing programs consider?

   a. Expenses of medical treatments
   b. Quality measures
   c. Procedures performed
   d. Quantity measures

90. Who contracts with CMS and serves as financial agents between the federal government and providers by performing prepayment reviews of locally administered Medicare Parts A and B medical claims?

   a. Medicare administrative contractor
   b. HHS Office of Inspector General
   c. Recovery audit contractor
   d. Document integrity specialist

91. A coding specialist uses computer-assisted coding software to code a patient's medical documentation. After reviewing the selected codes, the coder notices that two different codes (20612-RT and 20612-LT) have been generated for the procedure aspiration of a ganglion cyst of the wrist. The coder closely examined the medical record and found that the provider documented that this procedure was to be performed on the right wrist in the office note. However, the operative note stated that this procedure was performed on the left wrist. What is the best course of action for the coder to take based on these circumstances?

   a. Query the patient's provider to clarify if the procedure was performed on the left or right wrist before selecting a code.
   b. Call the floor the patient was on and ask the nurse which wrist the procedure was performed on.
   c. The coder should report both codes because each appears at least once in the medical documentation.
   d. Report the left wrist because it was documented in the operative note.

92. Mrs. Davis is preparing to undergo bariatric surgery but is required to obtain permission from her health insurer before receiving the procedure. What is the term used to describe this concept?

   a. Prior authorization
   b. Preapproval
   c. Preclearance
   d. Prior acceptance

93. Which of the following is a valuable data dictionary that serves as a resource for information system development?
    a. Passive data dictionary
    b. Organization-wide data dictionary
    c. DBMS data dictionary
    d. MPI data dictionary

94. A small medical practice is in the process of implementing an EHR system. The HIM director and IT department have agreed to use a strategy that allows everyone to go live at once and halt paper processing promptly after implementation. Based on this information, which rollout strategy does this describe?
    a. Parallel processing
    b. Straight turnover
    c. Phased rollout
    d. Go-live

95. A coding specialist has been assigning codes straight from the charge description master without using any human intervention. What is the term used to describe the actions of this coding specialist?
    a. Assumption coding
    b. Hard coding
    c. Soft coding
    d. Computer-assisted coding

96. Which of the following is NOT a component of the Resident Assessment Instrument in long-term care settings?
    a. Utilization Guidelines
    b. Care Area Assessments
    c. The Minimum Data Set
    d. Healthcare-associated infections

97. An organization is in the process of determining appropriate productivity standards for the billing department. The billing department's productivity standards must reflect what elements of the organization?
    a. Values and ethics
    b. Structure and finances
    c. Mission and goals
    d. Vision and values

98. A healthcare facility offers real-time, instructor-led online training that employees attend through an online learning platform. Which of the following best describes the training method offered?
    a. Synchronous
    b. Asynchronous
    c. Informal training
    d. E-learning

99. Which of the following is a standardized set of performance measures used to make comparisons of various managed health plans?

   a. UACDS
   b. HEDIS
   c. DEEDS
   d. RAVEN

100. Today, Olivia will undergo a hip replacement at Silver Pine Hospital. Who is responsible for obtaining Olivia's informed consent before the procedure is performed?

   a. An HIM professional
   b. Any medical professional
   c. The surgeon
   d. The administrative staff

101. A hospital has initiated peer reviews of medical providers' documentation to assess quality outcomes of care. This task can be overwhelming because the hospital currently employs more than 300 providers. It is eventually decided that 30% of each provider's discharge reports will be reviewed on an every-other-year basis. Which of the following techniques has this hospital applied to conduct its review process?

   a. Predictive methods
   b. Descriptive statistical analysis
   c. Sampling
   d. Benchmarking

102. A data analyst has asked you to help collect information about the effects that alcohol consumption has on people when they have the flu. You have been asked to collect the following information:

   - Whether or not a person has consumed any alcohol throughout the duration of their flu
   - How many hours of sleep occurred the night before
   - The person's temperature during the day that alcohol was consumed

What are the levels of measurement used for each data point?

   a. Nominal, ordinal, interval
   b. Ratio, interval, ordinal
   c. Interval, nominal, ratio
   d. Ordinal, interval, nominal

103. Edward has been tasked with bringing data from multiple sources into a centralized database. He wants to apply the most widely used data integration technique to manage big data. Based on this information, which of the following techniques should Edward choose?

   a. Manual data integration
   b. Change data capture
   c. Extract, transform, and load
   d. A record locator service

104. A hospital requires that all patient phone numbers be displayed in the following format: (XXX) XXX-XXXX. This format is an example of which of the following?
   a. Data definition
   b. Mask
   c. Structured data
   d. Wildcard

105. When revisions have to be made to clinical documentation, what is the proper way to make these corrections of medical record errors?
   a. Make the necessary corrections in the original medical record and authenticate the edits.
   b. Corrections of electronic medical records can never be made.
   c. Keep the record containing the error, create an entirely new medical record, and label it as a revised version.
   d. Delete the record containing the error before creating a new version of the medical record.

106. A patient who requested a copy of his medical record last week noticed a discrepancy in the documentation. He has asked that the erroneous information be corrected to avoid future medical errors. Which of the following terms is used to describe the changes made to correct the medical record in this instance?
   a. Alternation
   b. Modification
   c. Redisclosure
   d. Amendment

107. A patient who participated in a clinical trial last year would like to participate in a new clinical trial this year. The principal investigator already has a consent form signed by the patient from last year's clinical trial. What is the most appropriate action that should be taken to move forward?
   a. Have the patient sign a new consent form because compound authorization is prohibited in this situation.
   b. Apply last year's consent form for this year's clinical trial.
   c. The principal investigator only needs to get verbal consent from the patient.
   d. Begin the clinical trial first, and get the patient to sign a consent form at some point during the trial.

108. What would a data statistician use to find, retrieve, and use data?
   a. Primary data
   b. Metadata
   c. Secondary data
   d. Database

109. You have been asked to consolidate your organization's MPI. During this process, you have noticed that a patient is listed twice in the MPI—once under Robert M. Smith and again under Bob M. Smith. These MPI entries contain the same DOB, address, SSN, phone number, and all other demographic information. What is this common MPI data quality issue?
   a. Duplicate
   b. Overlay
   c. Repeat
   d. Overlap

110. Which of the following policies focuses on decision-making authority over data-related matters?
   a. Data modeling
   b. Data infrastructure
   c. Data analytics
   d. Data governance

111. An individual is permitted to access ePHI when belonging to a specific group, has a workstation located within a particular area within a facility, and possesses proper login and password credentials. Which security access mechanism would this individual be considered to have?
   a. Rule-based access control
   b. User-based access control
   c. Role-based access control
   d. Context-based access control

112. An individual has presented to your medical records department requesting an accounting of disclosures. According to the HITECH Act, an accounting of disclosures should include disclosures made over what period?
   a. The previous year
   b. The previous 3 years
   c. The previous 6 years
   d. The previous 10 years

113. A risk management department has just conducted a comprehensive HIPAA risk analysis and has to decide what measures to use to address uncovered risks. What are the three basic methods that the risk management department can implement?
   a. Avoid, mitigate, and transfer
   b. Mitigate, transfer, and accept
   c. Ignore, avoid, and transfer
   d. Prioritize, avoid, and accept

114. Which of the following is the most accurate definition of the National Health Information Network's Data Use and Reciprocal Support Agreement?
   a. A set of rules for patients to view and download their health records
   b. A legal agreement that defines requirements for the eHealth Exchange national network
   c. Requirements for covered entities to report breaches of unsecured PHI
   d. An HL7 XML-based document markup standard used for the electronic exchange of clinical documents

115. A healthcare professional has detected fraudulent activities occurring in his department. After bringing up this concern to his supervisor, he was discouraged from speaking about it any further and was immediately dismissed. This healthcare professional feels strongly about reporting these wrongdoings because they are ethically wrong. What is a term that this individual could be regarded as based on this information?
   a. Champion
   b. Informant
   c. *Qui tam relator*
   d. Corrupt employee

116. A hospital's data dictionary has included the following data descriptors regarding the data element ADMISSION_DATE: Definition, the date a patient was admitted to the hospital; data type, date; required field, yes; field length, 15; and acceptable values, none. To preserve data integrity, what change should be made to the data descriptors?
   a. Require a clearer data definition.
   b. Require a longer field length.
   c. Require acceptable data field values.
   d. Do not require this field.

117. The chief information officer (CIO) had a meeting with the IT department and suggested that the team take security initiatives by installing a network that uses a private tunnel through the internet, allowing more secure transmission of ePHI. The CIO claims that this network will help protect remote workers' connections. What type of network is the CIO referring to?
   a. Enterprise private network
   b. Wide-area network
   c. Virtual private network
   d. Local-area network

118. What is wrong with the following table?

Work Productivity of HIM Department		
RHIT	154	31.4
RHIA	372	68.6
Total	526	100.0

   a. The credential holder titles are inappropriate.
   b. The column totals are not correct.
   c. The use of decimals is not necessary.
   d. The column headings are missing.

119. Anne is a nurse requesting to see the medical records of her 21-year-old son who was hospitalized at the facility where she has been employed for the past 20 years. She is requesting medical records about an appendectomy her son had undergone 10 years ago. What is the appropriate action to take in this situation?
   a. Allow the nurse access because she is employed by the facility.
   b. Allow the nurse access because she is the son's guardian.
   c. Deny the nurse access because her son is now an adult and authorization from her son is required.
   d. Deny the nurse access because this document reached the end of its retention period and is no longer kept on file.

120. A doctor is curious about how many patients that he has treated have had cancer as a principal diagnosis over the past 2 years. Which index would be the best secondary data source for gathering this information?
   a. Disease index
   b. Physician index
   c. Operation index
   d. Master patient index

121. What term best describes the ability of various health IT systems and applications to work together through the precise and seamless exchange of information with one another?
   a. Effective communication
   b. Interoperability
   c. Interdisciplinarity
   d. Efficient electronic transitions

122. Which of the following options establishes a legally binding relationship between vendors and HIPAA-covered entities that entails specific requirements, such as prohibiting the use or disclosure of PHI if the subcontractors have potential access to this information?
   a. Physician service agreement
   b. Nondisclosure agreement
   c. Transfer agreement
   d. Business associate agreement

123. A healthcare provider inadvertently violates the HIPAA Privacy Rule in which of the following scenarios without explicit authorization from the patient(s) or their representative(s)?
   a. Reports sexually transmitted disease infection cases to the local health department.
   b. Sends birth statistics to the county registrar.
   c. Releases names and phone numbers of diabetic patients to a pharmaceutical company.
   d. Recommends a steroid to a patient with COPD.

124. Following a recent site survey, it has been determined that your healthcare organization has met The Joint Commission's requirements of the Conditions of Participation. Based on these results, your organization has earned which of the following?
   a. Certification authority
   b. Privileged communication
   c. Workforce clearance
   d. Deemed status

125. Upon reviewing a recent EHR audit, the HIM director discovers that an employee accessed the medical records of patients who share the same last name as the user multiple times. What is the most appropriate action to take in this situation?
   a. Terminate the employee immediately.
   b. Determine what information was accessed and why.
   c. Take no action because this is not a privacy issue.
   d. Revoke the employee's access rights.

126. Due to current staff shortages, two employees have been hired to complete a short-term coding project. These coders are hired through a third-party service that is out of the country and specializes in medical coding. What kind of alternate staffing method is this organization using?
   a. Flextime
   b. Outsourced
   c. Seasonal
   d. Job sharing

127. Sophia plays a significant role in her healthcare organization. She addresses inefficiencies in operations, assists with overcoming barriers, and promotes change. What term would be used to describe Sophia's innovative role?

a. Sponsor
b. Mentor
c. Critic
d. Champion

128. Recent flooding has occurred at a warehouse that stored medical records and has caused enough damage to require these documents to have to be moved to a new storage location. The majority of these records are at least 10 years old. What is the most appropriate course of action to take regarding the retention of these records before the move?

a. Ensure that the records are not involved in pending litigation or pertain to minors.
b. Destroy all of the records because 10 years have elapsed.
c. Decide how many records to keep based on the available storage at the new location.
d. Do not destroy any records; move them all to the new storage location.

129. A patient with diabetes mellitus is experiencing trouble managing her condition and the associated symptoms. This patient would like to meet more frequently with her physician but resides in a rural, underserved area, making travel difficult. What service could this patient use to conveniently meet with her physician without leaving home?

a. Videoconferencing
b. Telehealth
c. Patient portal
d. Personal health record

130. What is the term used to describe the probability of erroneously rejecting the null hypothesis when it is true?

a. T-test
b. F-ratio
c. Z-score
d. P-value

131. All of the following are examples of value-based care models EXCEPT:

a. Accountable care organizations
b. Patient-centered medical homes
c. Fee for service
d. Bundled payments

132. A provider has recently lost admission privileges due to incomplete medical records that have exceeded a specified time frame. What is the term used to describe these records?

a. Tardy records
b. Delinquent records
c. Overdue records
d. Delayed records

133. In a data governance program, what role is responsible for monitoring the data quality of the unit?

   a. Data stakeholders
   b. Data stewards
   c. Data analysts
   d. Data programmers

134. A specialty office that often treats highly complex patients has gotten in the habit of reporting the highest level of evaluation and management codes regardless of an individual's condition. What kind of fraudulent activity would this be considered?

   a. Unbundling
   b. Double billing
   c. Undercoding
   d. Upcoding

135. The local media and the secretary of HHS must be notified when the number of breached patient records is greater than or equal to what amount?

   a. 500
   b. 1,000
   c. 5,000
   d. 10,000

136. An HIM professional has begun organizing a database by breaking down data elements and creating entity relationship diagrams. This technique should eliminate redundancies and improve data quality. What is this process called?

   a. Normalization
   b. Elimination
   c. Expert determination
   d. Amortization

137. A patient has presented to your office with a confirmed case of mpox. What is the appropriate action that the office should take to report it?

   a. Send a letter reporting this case to the local health department.
   b. Immediately call and report this case to the local health department.
   c. Contact local hospitals to report this case.
   d. No action is required because this case does not need to be reported.

138. Use the table and graph provided to answer the question.

Coders	Status	Department
Kaleigh	Full-time	Emergency
Zoelle	Part-time	Outpatient
Daniel	Full-time	Inpatient
Hobart	Part-time	Inpatient

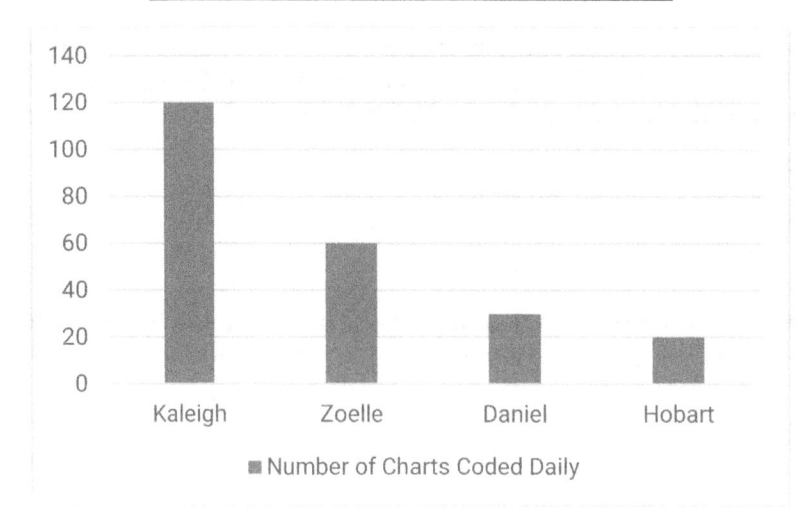

Number of Charts Coded Daily: Kaleigh 120, Zoelle 60, Daniel 30, Hobart 20

What conclusion can be made regarding the productivity of these four coders?
a. Kaleigh is the only coder meeting productivity standards.
b. There is not enough information to make a valid conclusion.
c. Hobart and Daniel are not working as hard as Kaleigh and Zoelle.
d. Hobart should be replaced because he is completing the lowest number of charts.

139. Recently, a data quality committee reviewed the inventory of its organization's databases as part of a newly implemented data integrity initiative. During the review, it was discovered that nearly half of the databases did not have an associated DBMS data dictionary. Based on these findings, what should be the first order of action for the committee to take?
a. Develop a training program for all workforce members on data dictionary use.
b. Send a memo to the workforce about the importance and value of a data dictionary.
c. Ignore the findings and focus efforts elsewhere.
d. Create a data dictionary policy and related standards.

140. Which of the following options allows HIE participants to search for records on the systems of other healthcare organizations' by using patient indexing and identification software?
a. Fee for service
b. Registry and directory service
c. Place of service
d. Record locator service

141. According to The Joint Commission, which document has to be placed into a patient's chart before any surgical procedure can be executed?

   a. Face sheet
   b. History and physical examination
   c. Advance directive
   d. Physician order

142. Which of the following is a standardized reporting system used to describe the performance of healthcare centers enabling comparisons for national benchmarks?

   a. Patient safety reporting system
   b. Clinical information system
   c. Uniform Data System
   d. Practice management system

143. During admission, a patient was given a Hospital-Issued Notice of Noncoverage (HINN) form. All of the following are valid reasons for a HINN to be provided EXCEPT:

   a. The service was custodial in nature.
   b. The service was not considered medically necessary.
   c. The service had not been preauthorized.
   d. The service was not delivered in the most appropriate setting.

144. An organization has budgeted $20,000 for a new industrial printer for the HIM department. The printer that was purchased cost $13,500. The excess capital would be referred to as what kind of accounting variance?

   a. Positive
   b. Favorable
   c. Good
   d. Superior

145. Leon, a data analyst, is extracting and filtering older data stored in various databases to see if he can discover any anomalies, trends, or correlations within the data set that have been missed or overlooked in the past. What is the activity that Leon is performing?

   a. Data sifting
   b. Data mining
   c. Data sorting
   d. Data mapping

146. Beth was just hired as a medical coder at a local hospital. She is informed that her first week will consist of orientation and shadowing others in her department. When can Beth expect to receive HIPAA compliance training?

   a. Only during her initial orientation period.
   b. After shadowing, when she begins working on her own.
   c. During orientation and throughout her employment with the hospital.
   d. She would not require HIPAA training for a coding position.

147. Abigail, an HIM professional, is the recipient of a *subpoena duces tecum*. What does this request require the healthcare professional to do?
   a. Conduct a deposition.
   b. Produce records at a proceeding.
   c. Serve as a jury member.
   d. Testify in court.

148. A patient was treated for three lacerations on the leg, all repaired with a simple closure. What would be the most appropriate CPT code for reporting in this situation?
   a. Use a single CPT code for the largest laceration.
   b. Use three CPT codes—one to report each laceration.
   c. Use a single CPT code to report the repair of the most complex closure.
   d. Use a single CPT code that sums all three lacerations together.

149. A physician ordered a chest x-ray for a patient who was complaining of leg pain. Based on this information, what is the clinical documentation lacking?
   a. Medical necessity
   b. Approved services
   c. Proper referral
   d. Family history

150. Mr. Brown's admission records indicate that his date of birth is November 23, 1956. However, Mr. Brown's date of birth on his discharge report is listed as November 23, 1965. What is the data quality element that is absent from Mr. Brown's medical record?
   a. Data granularity
   b. Data accuracy
   c. Data consistency
   d. Data relevancy

151. Following an automated recovery audit contractor review, a potential denial is flagged, and an alert is sent to encourage further evaluation. Which of the following examples would likely be denied and considered an improper payment without having access to the medical record documentation?
   a. Two appendectomies billed on the same day for the same patient
   b. Bilateral carpal tunnel procedure
   c. A principal procedure code
   d. A principal diagnosis code

152. All of the following would be considered necessary strategies to succeed when implementing value-based care EXCEPT:
   a. Charge for the quantity of services.
   b. Address any gaps in care.
   c. Leverage technology.
   d. Identify high-risk patients.

153. Mia has agreed to help employees navigate a newly installed EHR system at her facility. She received specialized training, was very involved in the EHR go-live date, possesses a deep understanding of the practice workflow, and offers to help troubleshoot when issues arise. What kind of user is Mia considered?

   a. Super user
   b. Remote user
   c. Database user
   d. Maintenance user

154. According to HIPAA's Privacy Rule, patients have the right to access, review, and receive a copy of their medical records for how long?

   a. As long as the records are maintained
   b. 6 years
   c. 10 years
   d. Indefinitely

155. After a coder reviews a patient's medical record, they create a physician query to clarify the patient's diagnosis. The documentation indicates the presence of a fever, body chills, and abdominal pain. Based on these symptoms, the coder assumes that a urinary tract infection (UTI) is present, although no urinalysis was conducted. Despite this, the coder asked the physician if they were treating the patient for a UTI. Based on this information, what option best represents what has occurred?

   a. Suggest adding a nonreportable diagnosis
   b. Increase reimbursement
   c. Closed-ended query
   d. Leading query

156. A doctor's office is reporting notifiable diseases in accordance with the CDC's National Notifiable Diseases Surveillance System. Which of the following would NOT fall under the category of notifiable diseases?

   a. Measles
   b. HIV infection
   c. Tetanus
   d. Diabetes mellitus

157. A medical coder has submitted the following CPT codes to capture a patient's recent procedure for billing purposes:

> **37760**—Ligation of perforator vein(s), subfascial, radical (Linton type) including skin graft, when performed, open (1 leg)
> **15271**—Application of skin substitute to trunk, arms, legs; total wound surface area up to 100 sq. cm; first 25 sq. cm or less wound surface area

Why was this claim denied?

   a. Underbilling
   b. Upcoding
   c. Unbundling
   d. Unfreezing

158. A healthcare organization is in the process of adding stronger physical safeguards within the facility. Which of the following would NOT be considered a form of physical safeguard according to the HIPAA Security Rule?

a. Locking doors to protected areas
b. Implementing security cameras
c. Using automatic logoff of computers
d. Installing smoke detectors and sprinklers

159. The infection prevention department created a summary report based on this year's trends of patients who have received the flu shot. What statement most accurately reflects the results of this report?

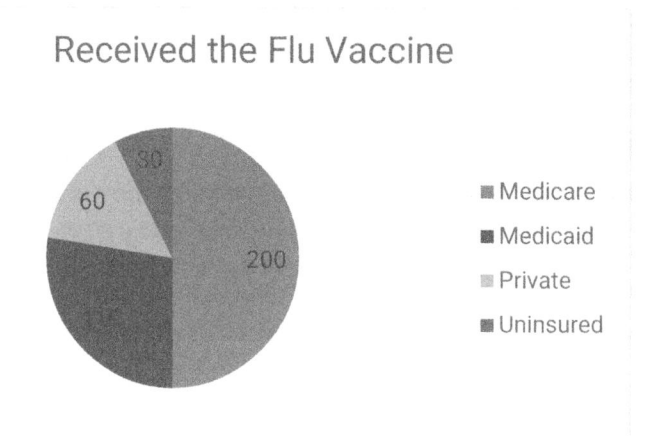

a. Uninsured patients do not want to get the flu vaccine.
b. The flu vaccine is mandated by health plans such as Medicare and Medicaid.
c. Medicare patients make up half of the individuals who have received the flu vaccine.
d. A patient's insurance status does not impact their ability to receive the flu vaccine.

160. You would like to verify the frequency distribution regarding the length of stay at your facility. What would be the best data display tool to use?

a. Dot plot
b. Bubble chart
c. Scatterplot
d. Histogram

161. A training program is being developed to educate staff on retention and destruction policies. The current lesson focuses on the actions taken following elapsed retention periods and the proper destruction of those medical records. After records are destroyed, a certificate of destruction is completed. How long should this document be retained by the facility?

a. 5 years
b. 10 years
c. 20 years
d. Permanently

162. Leah has been tasked with recruiting new employees. Which of the following best describes what she will be doing?
   a. Onboarding, training, and preparing new employees for the workplace.
   b. Finding, attracting, and evaluating potential new employees.
   c. Educating, mentoring, and supporting new employees on organizational policies/procedures.
   d. Collaborating, peer reviewing, and benchmarking new employees.

163. When a new employee is hired, they must complete an onboarding process before transitioning into their new position. What is the term that is used to describe this process?
   a. Admission
   b. Enrollment
   c. Orientation
   d. Training

164. What is the inpatient data set required for Medicare reporting?
   a. UHDDS
   b. OASIS
   c. HAVEN
   d. MDS

165. To ensure compliance with privacy initiatives, all covered entities and their business associates are required to train which workforce members?
   a. Only employees who have access to computer systems
   b. Only medical staff and nurses
   c. Administrative, medical, and IT staff members
   d. All workforce members throughout the organization

166. Which kind of technology focuses on data security, is situated between routers of private and public networks, and controls external access to a network?
   a. Firewall
   b. Encryptor
   c. Router
   d. Server

167. Of the options provided, which is a characteristic of the Breach Notification Rule?
   a. Notification should occur when an ROI specialist releases medical records to a patient after receiving a signed authorization form.
   b. Notification is only required when 500 or more individuals' PHI is affected.
   c. Local media must be notified following any unauthorized disclosure.
   d. When any individual's PHI has been breached, they must be notified.

168. A group of nurses is practicing realistic clinical scenarios for training purposes. This group can measure vital signs, place intravenous lines, and perform cardiopulmonary resuscitation in a lifelike environment without putting patients at risk. Which of the following is the training method that the nurses are using?
   a. Coaching
   b. Case studies
   c. Role-playing
   d. Simulations

169. A hospital's quality committee has collected data to assess the organization's performance. What conclusions can be made based on the following data regarding the hospital's quality of care in the third and fourth quarters?

Quality Measures	Third Quarter	Fourth Quarter
Patient falls	9.3%	4.6%
Adverse medication reactions	6.8%	3.4%
Wrong surgery site error	5.3%	1.9%
Hospital-acquired conditions	7.1%	2.5%

   a. The quality of care declined in the third and fourth quarters.
   b. The quality of care improved in the third and fourth quarters.
   c. The quality of care remains the same in the third and fourth quarters.
   d. The quality of care should not be determined on these measures.

170. A patient has high blood pressure with senile degeneration of the heart. What is the correct code selection?

> I10—Essential (primary) hypertension
> I51.5—Myocardial degeneration
> Fatty degeneration of the heart or myocardium
> Senile degeneration of the heart or myocardium
> I51.9—Heart disease, unspecified
> I95.0—Idiopathic hypotension

   a. I10, I95.0
   b. I10, I51.5
   c. I10, I51.9
   d. I51.5, I95.0

171. A quality team reviews medical records to determine if the information contained within the documentation is accurate and complete to improve the specificity of recorded medical conditions. What technique is the quality team performing?
   a. Continuity of care
   b. Clinical documentation improvement
   c. Causal-comparative research
   d. Chart conversion

172. An interdisciplinary team is responsible for undertaking an organization-wide initiative. The team is in the stage of the project in which discrepancies are resolved and they begin working together in harmony. What FSNP stage is this?

 a. Norming
 b. Forming
 c. Storming
 d. Performing

173. After compiling and analyzing data from various sources, a hospital has discovered that 25% of patients admitted to the facility have Medicaid as their primary insurance. What type of data is this an example of?

 a. Unstructured data
 b. Aggregate data
 c. Accession data
 d. Standardized data

174. What document must be issued to Medicare beneficiaries when an outpatient service is not likely to be covered by Medicare?

 a. Explanation of benefits (EOB)
 b. Advanced Beneficiary Notice of Noncoverage (ABN)
 c. Medicare summary notice (MSN)
 d. Remittance advice (RA)

175. A hospital has recently donated some of its computers to a local high school. A few of these computers still contained sensitive ePHI. What controls should the hospital use to minimize this kind of security breach from happening again?

 a. Role-based access controls
 b. Access controls
 c. Facility access controls
 d. Device and media controls

176. According to the value-based purchasing program, which statement about the total performance score (TPS) is most accurate?

 a. A higher TPS is preferable.
 b. The TPS does not matter in value-based purchasing.
 c. A lower TPS is preferable.
 d. A consistent TPS is preferable.

177. A physician has requested the medical record of a patient who has presented to the emergency department in critical condition. However, the patient's primary care physician has disabled the ability of his staff to share electronic health information with other healthcare systems. Based on this information, what has just occurred?

 a. Fraud
 b. Safe harbor method
 c. Information blocking
 d. Compliance with the HIPAA Privacy Rule

178. Leo is developing a comprehensive plan that addresses long-term needs based on his organization's mission, strengths, weaknesses, opportunities, and threats. What kind of plan is Leo creating?
   a. Operational plan
   b. Tactical plan
   c. Strategic plan
   d. Contingency plan

179. Which data visualization tool would be best to display nominal data that show the relative proportions and percentages of a whole data set?
   a. Pie chart
   b. Histogram
   c. Scatterplot
   d. Bar graph

180. Which of the following services detects and prevents coding and billing errors to reduce denied claims submitted to insurance companies?
   a. Cleaner
   b. Scrubber
   c. Encoder
   d. Grouper

181. Which of the following is essential information to incorporate in an MPI?
   a. Patient's name, vital signs, and phone number
   b. Patient's height, gender, and social security number
   c. Patient's disposition, weight, and discharge date(s)
   d. Patient's name, date of birth, and medical record number

182. Which HIE architectural model combines the functionality of a centralized data repository and a record locator service?
   a. Centralized
   b. Decentralized (federated)
   c. Consolidated
   d. Hybrid

183. An organization has recently implemented an MPI and needs to decide what information will be used to identify individuals. Which of the following is a unique identifier that should be used for the accurate identification of each patient?
   a. Patient address
   b. Patient date of birth
   c. Patient ID number
   d. Patient last name

184. All of the following are necessary components to include when developing policies and procedures for information governance EXCEPT:
   a. The scope of the policy or procedure
   b. Legalese used throughout
   c. The responsible parties involved
   d. Definitions of words and abbreviations

185. What purpose does an organization's practice management system serve?
    a. Allows clinicians to practice using health IT systems
    b. Manages the practice's medical staff
    c. Handles the training needs of staff in an organization
    d. Streamlines administrative and billing functions

186. Which system sends notifications on patients' status as they transition through various levels of care in a facility?
    a. Admit, discharge, and transfer system
    b. Electronic medical record
    c. Personal health record
    d. Practice management system

187. Which of the following is NOT a function of data governance?
    a. Conduct a one-time project to sort statistical data.
    b. Coordinate all of the data management domains.
    c. Organize and implement effective data management policies.
    d. Grant authority to certain individuals for data-related decisions.

188. An HIM professional has recently begun developing a record retention program for their organization. What legal source should the HIM professional defer to determine how long to retain medical records?
    a. State laws
    b. Joint Commission standards
    c. Hospital policies
    d. HIPAA retention guidelines

189. All of the following are matching algorithms used to detect and prevent instances of duplicate EMPI entries EXCEPT:
    a. Rules based
    b. Probabilistic
    c. Work based
    d. Deterministic

Answer Key and Explanations for Test #2

1. A: System configuration is an essential step of information technology (IT) system implementation, which focuses on making a system or software application work for a particular organization. System configuration usually begins with assessments of the organization's infrastructure and ability to support the new system. It can also consist of adapting and aligning technical components to support workflows. Adjusting decision support rules, customizing screens, writing interfaces, and implementing measures to meet privacy and security compliance can all be considered vital components of system configuration.

2. D: Performing audit trails helps to reconstruct electronic events to maintain the privacy of patients. Audit controls are considered a category of technical safeguards that include the technology and policies/procedures used to protect electronic protected health information (ePHI). Curious workforce members may conduct unauthorized searches of the celebrity patient's medical records and may even leak or try to sell this information for attention or personal gain. Therefore, healthcare organizations must ensure that additional security precautions are taken to protect the confidentiality of public figures.

3. B: A fishbone diagram, also known as a cause-and-effect or Ishikawa diagram, is a visualization tool used to determine and explore all of the possible causes of a problem. This tool is often used during the analysis phase of Six Sigma's define, measure, analyze, improve, and control (DMAIC) approach. The problem is placed in a box at the far-right side of the diagram, a line is drawn from the problem, and approximately 4–6 primary categories (i.e., methods, manpower, machines, materials, measurements, and more) that contribute to the problem are placed in boxes connected to the problem line. Diagonal lines also stem from each cause box containing secondary and possibly tertiary issues related to that category. This analysis assists with determining the ultimate root cause of a problem.

4. A: Covered entities are obligated under the Health Insurance Portability and Accountability Act of 1996 (HIPAA) to allow individuals to make specific privacy requests; however, they are not always required to honor the patient's request. For example, if a patient pays for a service in full out of pocket, they have the right to restrict disclosures of PHI regarding this service. This special request must be in writing, and a signed copy should be kept if the covered entity agrees to the request.

5. C: According to the Joint Commission, operative reports must be written, dictated, and entered into the medical record immediately after surgery of a high-risk procedure. If an operative report cannot be completed, a progress note must be entered before the patient is transferred to the next level of care to ensure that pertinent information is available to subsequent caregivers.

6. C: Movement diagrams visually depict a workspace layout that includes doorways, furniture, equipment workstations, and more. The movements of daily work can be traced to examine inefficiencies in workflow processes. Equipment and workstations can be rearranged for process improvement purposes that could result in smoother and more effective office workflows.

7. C: The capitated rate is also known as per member per month (PMPM) or per patient per month (PPPM). This payment method refers to physicians providing all contracted healthcare services to a group of patients and reimbursing a fixed amount for each individual. For example, a doctor could be reimbursed $150 per patient per month. A practice with 50 enrolled members would be compensated a total of $7,500 per month regardless of whether all patients were seen during this period.

8. A: A job description is a written explanation used to outline and clearly define the work performed by a person in a specific job position. Other information that can be found in job descriptions includes, but is not limited to, working conditions, skills/competency requirements, and the individual to whom the employee(s) must report.

9. D: The chief complaint refers to the principal reason or symptoms that a patient is experiencing that caused the patient to seek medical care as told in the patient's own words. In this scenario, the patient presented to the facility complaining of a severe headache. Therefore, this would be considered the chief complaint.

10. D: The analyze, design, develop, implement, evaluate (ADDIE) model is a flexible, systematic framework used to develop training programs. ADDIE uses a cyclical approach to create training/education programs. Below is a breakdown of this process.

- Analyze the organization and perform a needs assessment.
- Design the curriculum based on objectives, learning methods, and techniques that will be used.
- Develop the curriculum and perform pilot tests to evaluate the program.
- Implement the program and schedule the training rollout.
- Evaluate the effectiveness of the training program, provide feedback, and make necessary adjustments.

11. A: A quality data dictionary should define the name, type (date, text, number, etc.) length, and values allowed to be used in each data field. Clear definitions for each data field or column should also be incorporated. Some other descriptors that may be included are data format, whether the field is required, and edits placed on the data fields. Although data dictionaries can be used during the process of database design, it is not necessary to include entity relationship diagrams regarding the data fields/columns in the data dictionary.

12. C: The problem-oriented medical record (POMR) is comprised of a problem list, initial plan, and progress notes so other professionals can easily follow the course of a person's treatment. The most recognizable component of the POMR is the use of the subjective, objective, assessment, plan (SOAP) format to document progress notes. This record format is commonly used by physicians or other healthcare providers who furnish treatment services to patients.

13. B: If the HIM director is only considering the retention period required by Medicare's Conditions of Participation (CoP), it would be most appropriate to retain this record until at least March 10, 2015. According to the CoP, medical records must be retained and be legally reproducible for at least 5 years.

14. C: The Stark Law, also known as the physician self-referral statute, prohibits physicians from referring patients for designated health services to any entities that the physician has a financial relationship with or who is an immediate family member. Designated health services can include, but are not limited to, clinical laboratory services, physical or occupational therapy, durable medical equipment, home health services, and outpatient prescription drugs.

15. B: When comparing the data to the information displayed in the graph, we can see that the values for the "wrong drug" and "wrong dose" should be switched. This mistake could have occurred during the creation of the summary report. A simple error in data input could result in the risk management team focusing its efforts on the wrong issues. This example demonstrates how close attention to detail is extremely important when summarizing data.

16. A: A swimlane diagram is very similar to a flowchart, except the diagram is broken up into lanes that delineate the individual(s) or group(s) responsible for a specific task. Each task is connected by arrows that signify the order of information or flow of a process. This cross-sectional flowchart allows for simultaneous viewing of everyone involved in a process. Swimlane diagrams are used to troubleshoot problems, standardize work processes, improve efficiency, and clarify accountability.

17. D: The Emergency Medical Treatment and Active Labor Act (EMTALA) is also referred to as the antidumping statute. EMTALA ensures that the public can receive emergency medical services regardless of ability to pay. EMTALA applies to hospitals that have provider agreements and accept payments from the Centers for Medicare and Medicaid Services (CMS) under the Medicare program. This act requires a patient's condition to be stabilized before transferring them another facility.

18. C: Six Sigma encompasses a set of management techniques intended to improve business processes. Define, measure, analyze, improve, and control (DMAIC) is the standard data-driven Six Sigma methodology used to reduce the number of defects in processes. The five phases are described below.

- Define the problem and the improvement opportunity.
- Measure performance.
- Analyze performance to determine the root causes of variances.
- Improve the process by addressing the root causes.
- Control the improved process.

19. C: The return on investment for an individual purchase can be calculated by dividing the earnings from the purchase by the total asset amount.

Step 1—Divide the earnings by the total assets:

$$\$36,000 \div \$150,000 = 0.24$$

Step 2—Multiply the decimal by 100 to get a percentage:

$$ROI = 0.24 \times 100 = 24\%$$

20. C: Copy-and-paste functionality allows users to duplicate information from a previous patient encounter to another. Although this practice is permitted, it should be used with caution because it can result in confusion, liability issues, redundancies in medical documentation, difficulties identifying the author, and the content copied and pasted may be outdated or inaccurate. Detailed policies and procedures should be created and maintained to monitor the appropriate use of the copy-and-paste functionality.

21. C: The HIPAA Privacy Rule addresses timely responses to requests for PHI. Covered entities and the individual(s) responsible for the release of medical records must respond to an individual's request no later than 30 days after the request has been made. In the event that medical records would take longer to retrieve—possibly due to being stored at an off-site location—the covered entity may be allowed to extend the request to 60 days. The requestor should be informed of the reason for the delay and should be provided with the date that the request will be fulfilled.

22. C: Coordination of benefits is a term used to describe the method used in determining which health insurance carrier is the primary payer and which one is the secondary payer when an individual has coverage through multiple insurers. (Medicaid will always be considered the payer of last resort.)

23. D: According to the official ICD-10-CM coding guidelines, codes presented in brackets should always be sequenced second. This coding convention instructs coders to first code any underlying disease or condition followed by the etiology or manifestations.

24. D: Structured Query Language (SQL) is the formal programming language used to sort, process, retrieve, update, and delete information in relational databases. Various SQL commands can be used to communicate with databases and assist with creating, manipulating, and accessing data across numerous tables.

25. D: Every healthcare organization should closely examine internal and external regulations to help shape its data governance programs. Considering external regulations helps ensure that data will be kept, maintained, and used in accordance with federal and state laws and can avoid noncompliance issues.

26. C: When healthcare professionals are granted licensure (which is issued on a statewide level), they have legal authorization to practice their occupation. Licensure is awarded to individuals when they show that they can meet industry- or state-approved quality standards by passing an examination. This ensures that professionals are proficient by meeting specific qualifications and continuing to maintain competencies in that given content area.

27. C: When conducting a SWOT analysis, opportunities may include ways to improve the business. An organization may assess its internal and external environments to try and determine how it may expand its operations, better leverage technology, or discover how other resources can be taken advantage of to enhance business operations or outcomes.

28. A: The net income is based on the arithmetic difference between total revenue and total expenses of the current fiscal year. Therefore, to calculate net income, you must subtract the total revenue from total expenses:

$$\$3,500,500 - \$2,000,500 = \$1,500,000$$

29. D: The custodian of medical records has various responsibilities related to legal proceedings such as appropriately releasing information to a designated recipient (typically an attorney), ensuring that requests for PHI are valid, and determining which portions of the medical record may be released. Another role that the custodian would be responsible for is testifying as to whether the records are admissible to admit as evidence.

30. D: The conflict management style used by the HIM manager in this scenario is accommodation. This resolution can occur when one party sacrifices a desired outcome to satisfy the other party. The accommodating style only works when one party is not invested as strongly in the conflict/outcome as the other. This allows the issue to be resolved more quickly and avoids prolonged conflict.

31. A: In general, healthcare providers (i.e., attending physicians) who are treating patients bear the responsibility of ensuring the quality of medical documentation. These individuals record the diagnoses, treatment, medical history, procedures performed, and other pertinent details that could be used in future medical decision-making processes.

32. C: A retrospective review is a cost-effective way to collect and analyze data after a patient is discharged from a healthcare facility. The goal of retrospective reviews is to determine if the patient's health benefits and member eligibility are correct and whether coverage after treatment has been given.

33. B: Based on the options listed, the correct CPT code for posterior arthrodesis of 7 vertebral segments with a cast is 22802. The other answer options are incorrect because code 22800 only covers up to 6 vertebral segments and codes 22808 and 22810 should be used for anterior spinal deformities.

34. A: Of the options listed in this question, two instances would not require a signed authorization form to obtain medical records on behalf of another individual. The caretaker of an incompetent adult patient can receive copies of the patient's medical records without the signed authorization of that patient. The patient (when competent) should, however, be given an opportunity in advance to agree or object to this individual being directly involved with their care in the event they can no longer care for themselves. The guardian(s) of a minor can also obtain their child's medical records without having to sign an ROI authorization form.

35. C: Record retention programs generally consist of conducting an inventory of the facility's records, determining the format and location of record storage, assigning each record a specific time for preservation, and destroying records only after they have reached the end of their retention period.

36. B: Shortages of healthcare workers can be alleviated by cross-training competent employees to perform the job of several team members. These employees can build a broader skill set and float to cover areas needing assistance. Cross-training affords flexibility in shifting workloads/resources and is most useful when work teams are involved.

37. A: After reviewing the data set, one disadvantage of using the mean length of stay as a facility statistic in this scenario is that it contains an outlier. Outliers that are present in a data set can skew the mean. For example, the values 3, 3, 4, 5, 6, 7, and 28 result in an average of 8. However, this value is on the high end of the data set because the outlier (28) has skewed the mean value. Therefore, based on the data presented, the median (5) would provide a more accurate measure of the facility's length of stay.

38. D: A scatterplot is a data analysis tool used to uncover relationships between two continuous variables. A line of best fit can be drawn between the middle of the points on the plot and is used to represent trends in the data. An ascending line is interpreted as a positive association, and a descending line represents a negative association. Therefore, this scatterplot shows a positive correlation between the increase of a patient's age and their likelihood of falling.

39. D: Based on the results of the employee turnover summary report, the performance improvement team should examine the cause of the high turnover rate in year 4. Years 1–3 are all much lower than year 4 which displays turnover rates higher than the internal and external benchmarks. The performance improvement team may be able to determine what the cause of the turnover rate is and use this as an opportunity for improvement.

40. B: Productivity standards provide a measure of performance expectations that should be based on volume and accuracy. These data are often used to justify the need for extra staff or equipment.

The following formula can be used to determine how many more pages per hour are required to meet productivity standards:

$$174 \text{ pages filed (per hour)} \div 0.50 = 348 \text{ pages}$$

$$348 \text{ pages} - 174 \text{ pages} = 174 \text{ additional pages}$$

Therefore, an additional 174 pages should be filed per hour for the HIM department to meet productivity standards.

41. B: The Latin term *stare decisis* means "let the decision stand." This principle refers to the legal doctrine of judicial precedence, in which state courts look at similar past issues that have been ruled on to guide decisions. Considering the ruling in previous historical cases helps to ensure uniform justice and fairness in similar legal cases or closely related issues.

42. D: Although contracts can vary in length, complexity, and terms, they all must contain essential elements that make them valid and legally enforceable. These elements often include, but are not limited to, an offer, acceptance, consideration, a mutual obligation, capacity, and legality.

43. B: Bugs are programming mistakes or source code errors that could affect a software application's performance by causing a program to crash or produce unexpected results. Although computer bugs could be considered a vulnerability to the facility's systems, they would not be considered malware.

44. C: Privileged communication, or physician–patient privilege, is a concept often delineated by state law, which is designed to protect confidentiality between two parties. Providers have an ethical duty to keep the communications between themselves and their patients private and must not improperly disclose details of an individual's private affairs.

45. B: Budget, scope, and schedule are all core project constraints that must be continuously monitored to avoid project failure. Other project constraints include risk, resources, and quality. The success of a project is determined by its ability to manage these constraints.

46. A: Administrative data are crucial for healthcare organizational operations that are associated with healthcare encounters. In order to run smoothly and efficiently, organizations must ensure that accurate documentation is kept on all patients and encounters. Administrative data may consist of patient demographics, enrollment, claims/eligibility data, and more.

47. B: The removal method should not be assumed, and the best course of action would be to ask the physician who performed the procedure about which method was used. It could be possible that multiple techniques were used to remove multiple polyps. In this case, modifier 59 (distinct procedural service) could be attached to bundled codes to receive appropriate reimbursement.

48. B: The Privacy Rule allows covered entities to charge reasonable cost-based fees associated with the function of release of PHI. These charges consider costs for labor, supplies used for making photocopies, and postage if the records are to be mailed (the price for these activities varies from state to state). However, patients are not always charged these fees. Typically, the covered entity will provide copies of PHI free of charge.

49. C: Healthcare providers send out superbills (detailed, itemized receipts distributed to patients and their insurance carriers). Other names used for this document include claim form, encounter form, charge slip, and fee ticket. The information on a superbill includes, but is not limited to, a patient's name, insurance information, diagnosis and procedure codes, date(s) of service, the provider's National Provider Identifier number, and any associated charges.

50. A: The accession number is used to identify patients in a cancer registry; the list of cases is arranged in the order in which they were entered. The first two digits represent the year when the patient was first seen at the facility. The remaining digits would be assigned sequentially throughout the year. In this example, the accession number reveals that the patient was first seen in 2004.

51. C: Incidence rates are used to compare the number of new cases of specific diseases over a given period to the population at risk for the disease during the same period. In this scenario, the 45 new cases of respiratory syncytial virus, compared to the entire pediatric population during a specific time, represents the incidence rate.

52. A: HIM professionals are responsible for validating ROI requests and determining whether access and disclosures of PHI are appropriate. HIM professionals apply their extensive knowledge of state and federal laws to ensure that ROI processes promote patient access rights while balancing the protection of their privacy.

53. D: The National Correct Coding Initiative (NCCI) is a program developed by CMS that is designed to promote correct coding methods and reduce improper Medicare Part B and Medicaid payments. Outpatient code editors are software programs linked to NCCI that apply logical rules to determine various combinations of procedures and services that cannot be billed together on the same day.

54. A: The Federal Trade Commission (FTC) created the Red Flag Rule to help organizations detect and prevent fraud. This rule requires organizations to implement an identity theft prevention program with corresponding policies and procedures to identify red flags. The ability to detect suspicious activities quickly during day-to-day operations can help mitigate damage and combat fraudulent actions. Information that does not match what your practice has on file such as a person's date of birth, social security number, or differences in a person's physical appearance would be considered a red flag and should be more closely examined.

55. C: The success of an EHR system can be dependent on physicians adopting and properly using this technology. If physicians complain that the system's interface is not user-friendly and exploring all its functionalities would be too time-consuming, it would be best to provide support staff and implement training programs for physicians. Explaining how healthcare technologies can improve patient care, help meet compliance standards, and make workflows more efficient might help influence physicians. Interfaces can be configured to make the navigation of EHRs easier. Also, providing support staff can aid throughout the training period and beyond.

56. C: All individuals have the right to revoke their consent for use and disclosure (in writing). However, if a covered entity has already released PHI in good faith based on the prior authorization of the patient, it would be covered under the Privacy Rule.

57. C: Patients who suspect that they are victims of identity theft can file a complaint with the FTC. This agency is responsible for the oversight of identity theft regulations. It offers support and comprehensive educational materials for consumers and victims.

58. C: In this scenario, Mr. Jones will be denied access to his wife's medical records. Generally, HIPAA does not allow the release of PHI to any individuals except for the patient without proper authorization. This includes the patient's friends, family members, spouse, or other loved ones. The exception to this rule is if the individual requesting PHI is the patient's caregiver or the patient has signed a HIPAA-compliant authorization form that specifies the individual to receive copies of medical records on behalf of the patient. Therefore, in this scenario, the office will require written authorization for the release of medical records signed by Bethany that designates her husband as being authorized to obtain a copy of her medical record. This should identify the range of approved disclosure, for example, if her spouse only receives copies of PHI in this instance or all records over a given period of time. It is recommended that this form be updated often to avoid breaches of privacy.

59. B: The revenue cycle has three distinct phases, including front-end, middle, and back-end processes. Front-end processes include scheduling, prior authorization, insurance verification, financial counseling, and more. The middle process involves charge capture, coding, clinical documentation, and case management. Back-end processes include claims processing, denial management, follow-ups, posting of payments, and collections.

60. A: The weight of each Medicare severity diagnosis related group (MS-DRG) should be multiplied by the number of discharges for that MS-DRG.

Step 1—Multiply each weight by the number of discharges:

$$1.2468 \times 20 = 24.936$$
$$0.6527 \times 20 = 13.054$$
$$0.9362 \times 10 = 9.362$$

Step 2—Sum the totals from step 1:

$$24.936 + 13.054 + 9.362 = 47.352$$

Step 3—Sum the total discharges:

$$20 + 20 + 10 = 50$$

Step 4—Divide the total weights by the total volume of discharges:

$$CMI = 47.352 \div 50 = 0.94704$$

61. C: Offering a variety of training methods can help meet the needs of individuals with different learning styles. Organizations that create an inclusive EHR training program combining techniques from each of the following learning styles have the potential to engage the largest number of their diverse workforce:

- Auditory learners—benefit from listening to lectures and audiobooks
- Visual learners—benefit from viewing visual content such as photos or videos
- Kinesthetic learners—use a hands-on approach to learn content
- Reading learners—absorb information best when they read about it

62. B: The information provided in this scenario—persistent registration errors despite implementing a new patient registration system—would infer that underlying human processes were not addressed and corrected beforehand. It is unlikely that both the new and old systems would result in the same registration errors. A closer examination of the department's workflow might uncover problems that could be addressed before implementing new health IT systems to solve the issue.

63. C: A legal hold requires carefully tracked handling of patient records involved in litigation. The special care and attention given to these records ensure that no changes can be made to these documents and protect them from being improperly destroyed or tampered with. This documentation must be preserved because it may serve as evidence in legal proceedings.

64. D: The compliance officer is conducting a focused audit of this specific coder's claims, on a retrospective basis. The only way to determine why these claims were denied is to compare the assigned codes to the medical documentation to verify the information. Performing this focused audit can better uncover error patterns, can be used to educate the coder, and will ultimately result in code/reimbursement optimization by decreasing instances of denied claims.

65. D: The HIPAA Privacy Rule allows healthcare facilities to maintain facility directories that can disclose basic information including a patient's location in the facility, and it can describe their condition is general terms to anyone who specifically asks for a patient by name. Patients have the right to opt out of a facility directory by filling out a form and can opt back in at any time. When a patient opts out of the directory, staff must not share any information regarding the patient's condition or location within the facility even if a family member is asking.

66. C: Barcoded medication administration (BCMA) technology has been implemented to assist in reducing human errors. Barcodes consist of arrangements of parallel dark bars and light spaces that can be located on patient wristbands, medication labels, specimen containers, or other records/items. Barcoding interprets data for identification and data collection purposes. In addition to reducing medication errors, barcoding technology can streamline billing and can be used to manage inventory.

67. D: The goal of performing a criticality analysis is to recognize how valuable an asset is to a business. An addressable requirement of the HIPAA Security Rule is to evaluate all systems/applications used by an organization to assess potential risks and determine the impacts that they could have on the business. This process is vital to data management and can be helpful in quickly restoring critical systems following expected or unexpected downtime.

68. B: A patient portal offers individuals 24-hour access to all or part of their medical records maintained by their healthcare provider. These portals are secure and require users to enter a username and password to view information from anywhere with an internet connection. Patient portals can also be used for requesting prescription refills, scheduling appointments, and accessing educational material.

69. D: Deploying questionnaire surveys is a way to query end users about their current use of EHR applications. Participants' responses can be used to make adjustments or improvements. Questionnaire surveys are a more cost- and time-effective option compared to conducting interviews. The survey may ask if users thought they were adequately trained, if they receive technical support when necessary, if they find the EHR easy to navigate, and if they are satisfied with their overall experience. The survey can also ask for users' opinions and comments on what changes could be made to improve the EHR system's effectiveness.

70. B: It is essential to conduct an ongoing maintenance program to ensure low rates of MPI quality issues. This process is often referred to as MPI or EMPI cleanup, which consists of using algorithms to detect dirty patient data. MPI cleanup efforts result in a reduction of redundant and inconsistent entries, help standardize data, and ensure data integrity.

71. A: The ruling on the *Tarasoff v. Regents of the University of California* case of 1976, held that mental health professionals have a duty to protect those threatened with bodily harm by a patient and have a responsibility to warn of the potential dangers that their patients could pose to others. The duty to warn can also extend to sexually transmitted diseases. Physicians may be held liable if they fail to warn third parties of any potential serious threats that could place them at risk.

72. C: A review of records completed while the patient is still in the facility is referred to as a concurrent, or open-record, review. This process is done to ensure that medical documentation is complete and that signatures of providers are present; it also helps determine if the diagnosis codes selected accurately support what is found in the medical record documentation. Any problems revealed during this process can be corrected immediately, thereby contributing to a better quality of care and improved health outcomes.

73. B: Bar graphs can be used to compare various groups or track significant changes over time. Data that are being tracked over a period of time would usually be better presented on a line plot.

74. A: The Logical Observations Identifier Names and Codes (LOINC) is a clinical terminology used to provide a common language, exchange standard, and mapping mechanism for laboratory test orders and results. Each LOINC code provides a detailed description of the laboratory tests ordered/completed, and the resulting data are displayed in a structured format.

75. A: A request for proposal (RFP) involves carefully researching specifications of technology desired by an organization. Because health IT systems are significant investments, organizations must exercise due diligence and ensure that potential vendors can meet their contractual specifications. The RFP uses a structured document that compels candidates to answer various questions that will be scored. RFPs are typically sent to four to six vendors. After scoring questions and conducting an internal review of potential vendors, the list will usually be narrowed down to three to four vendors. Internal interviews will outline clear expectations by the requesting organization, demonstrations of vendors' products, and reference checks. Site visits provide a better understanding of the vendors and their products. This allows an organization to compare primary functionality, user-friendliness, and potential downfalls of multiple systems before making a decision.

76. A: The breach at facility 1 would be considered a tier 3 violation because the category falls under willful neglect, but the facility corrected the violation within 30 days after its discovery. The penalty for this type of breach can range from $10,000 to $50,000 per violation. If the facility had not corrected the violation after 30 days, it would be considered a tier 4 violation.

77. D: Authentication is the process of identifying the author who created an entry in a medical record and attesting that it is genuine. The use of a password, a handwritten or digital signature, or biometric identifiers can establish the user who originated the documentation. All entries in health records must be authenticated to provide verification of the author's identity.

78. A: The tracer methodology is a technique used by on-site Joint Commission surveyors that can identify performance or process issues. The tracer methodology is often conducted by following the experience of care, treatment, and services rendered to selected patients. It can also be used to assess operational systems.

79. B: Covered entities must report breaches of PHI to the secretary of HHS, in addition to informing the affected individuals. According to HIPAA's Breach Notification Rule, for breaches affecting up to 500 individuals, a covered entity must notify the secretary of HHS no later than 60 days after the end of the calendar year when the breach was discovered. A breach report form can be found on the HHS website and should be filled out and submitted by the covered entity.

80. D: Vocabulary standards support data integrity by implementing common and consistent definitions for medical concepts or characterization of a patient's condition. Using uniform vocabulary standards helps enhance reporting, improve quality, and assist with interoperability for the effective exchange of health information.

81. A: Benefits, payroll, and office supplies cover some of the day-to-day expenses and focus on projected income statement activity spanning 1 fiscal year. On the other hand, large-dollar purchases/investments such as office equipment (computers, printers, office furniture, etc.) would be included in a capital budget. Capital acquisitions may span from 1 to 3 years.

82. A: The correct ICD-10-PCS code for cryoablation of skin lesion on the right breast would be 0H5TXZZ. The section is medical and surgical, the body system is skin and breast, the root operation is destruction, the body part is right breast, an external approach would be used, and no device or qualifier is required.

83. A: A notice of privacy practices is a document that describes the duty the healthcare entity has to protect healthcare information privacy, informs patients of their own privacy rights, and notifies them of how their PHI may be used or shared by their health plan or provider under the HIPAA Privacy Rule. The notice of privacy practices must provide examples of PHI uses/disclosures that are permitted or required for treatment, payment, and healthcare operations and for other purposes. Patients will be asked to sign an acknowledgment of receipt of this notice.

84. A: The HIPAA Privacy Rule requires special protections for psychotherapy notes. Psychotherapy notes are a treating provider's personal notes kept separate from the medical record that contain sensitive information regarding a provider's opinion on a patient. These notes are often used to help the therapist recall details of sessions and are not typically shared with other healthcare professionals. The exceptions for disclosures of psychotherapy notes (when required by law) include reporting abuse or instances of duty to warn when a patient makes threats to harm another individual. However, patients have the right to access their mental health records, and an ROI specialist could release the records after confirming with the physician that it would not be considered harmful to the patient.

85. D: The HIM professional should inform the employer that signed authorization from the patient is required before any medical records can be released. To protect the patient's privacy, only the minimum necessary information should be released to the employer to accomplish their intended purposes. Be aware that in some states, employers, their attorneys, or their insurers may not require patient authorization to obtain the minimum necessary PHI of that individual for workers' compensation purposes.

86. B: Statistical techniques such as decision trees, logistic regressions, and cluster analyses are all visualization tools used in predictive modeling to create models to assess the probability of fraudulent claims.

- Decision trees can create characteristics or profiles of fraudulent behaviors so these cases can be extracted and examined more closely.
- Logistic regressions help predict expected claim values and identify cases that fall outside the expected range.
- Cluster analyses can be used to group a provider's transactions and perform outlier identification by using association algorithms.

87. C: A review of systems is a structured technique that physicians use to keep an inventory of a patient's body systems by asking the individual a series of questions to identify any possible symptoms the patient may be experiencing. CMS recognizes 14 body systems that include, but are not limited to, gastrointestinal, genitourinary, musculoskeletal, neurological, psychiatric, endocrine, and allergic/immunologic.

88. D: A physician query is a communication and education tool used to seek clarification on clinical documentation or to gain further specificity regarding patient care. A standardized query process is typically developed in each healthcare organization to increase the precision of medical documentation. Medical coders use this process to question the physician who created the medical record and include supporting information captured in the documentation.

89. B: A value-based purchasing program reimburses quality instead of the quantity of care provided. The goal is to promote the triple aim (improving individuals' experiences, enhancing population health, and reducing healthcare costs). A hospital's performance will be based on quality measures that impact reimbursement rates.

90. A: Medicare administrative contractors (MACs) are awarded geographic jurisdiction to process Medicare Parts A and B claims. They perform prepayment reviews to ensure services are considered medically necessary and are covered. Other MAC duties include, but are not limited to, educating providers, establishing local coverage determinations, coordinating with CMS and other contractors, and handling the appeals process.

91. A: Inconsistencies in clinical documentation often result in poor patient outcomes, improper reimbursement, medical errors, and much more. Therefore, when medical records consist of conflicting information, the best way to request clarification is to use the communication tool known as a physician query. In this situation, the coder should query the provider who created the documentation before reporting any codes.

92. A: Prior authorization, or precertification, occurs when a physician obtains permission from the patient's insurance carrier to provide certain services. This process is often done to ensure that the services provided meet medical necessity standards and would be covered under the beneficiary's healthcare plan.

93. B: An organization-wide data dictionary helps drive data standards while promoting consistency and quality across the entire organization. This data dictionary serves as a valuable resource for information system development because it can assist technologists and organizational leaders in understanding the enterprise terms and their definitions to better use consumer data.

94. B: The most common form of EHR turnover is straight turnover. This rollout method takes a big-bang approach and is typically used by smaller organizations. Straight turnover is designed so everyone in the designated group will go live at one time. Immediately after the go-live date, the processing of paper documents should cease because it can be time-consuming and veers away from meaningful use of the EHR system. However, temporary paper processing might be necessary for a short time until users can process electronic information correctly.

95. B: Hard coding refers to the coding of repetitive or noncomplex services using the CDM without human intervention. Hard coding could also include delegating coding responsibilities to individuals who are not coding specialists and are not familiar with coding guidelines. Soft coding requires the knowledge and intervention of a coding professional who assesses the clinical documentation to assign diagnosis or procedure codes. Although both methods may be used in healthcare facilities, soft coding is the recommended practice—hard coding should be avoided.

96. D: The Minimum Data Set, Care Area Assessments, and Utilization Guidelines are all components of the Resident Assessment Instrument in long-term care settings. Together, these three elements furnish information regarding a resident's preferences and functional status, while providing additional guidance concerning future assessments after issues have been identified. Although healthcare-associated infections may be tracked in long-term care, they are not a component of the Resident Assessment Instrument.

97. C: Productivity standards should be aligned with an organization's mission and goals and can be used to guide the actions and behaviors of the workforce. Goals should be specific, measurable, actionable, realistic, and timely to increase the likelihood of reaching and even boosting productivity standards.

98. A: Synchronous training refers to real-time gatherings of instructors and learners that can occur virtually or physically. This type of training allows instantaneous communication, collaboration, and the ability for instructors to address questions or concerns as they arise. Although disadvantages can include scheduling conflicts, learning is set at the instructor's pace, and students may not receive individual attention.

99. B: The Healthcare Effectiveness Data and Information Set (HEDIS) was developed by the National Committee for Quality Assurance. HEDIS supplies healthcare consumers and purchasers with the information that is required to compare the performance of managed healthcare plans. More than 70 measures—compared to national or regional benchmarks—are used to assess the quality of healthcare plan services delivered.

100. C: Invasive procedures or treatments that may be considered risky should not be performed until informed consent is obtained from the patient. The provider responsible for performing the procedure should obtain the patient's consent. The surgeon should attempt to answer any questions from the patient regarding the procedure and must detail the nature of the service, outline the expected benefits and risks, provide alternative treatment options, and explain the possible consequences of not performing the procedure.

101. C: It would be a difficult and time-consuming task to assess even a handful of records from each provider. The hospital can, however, use the sampling technique to randomly select and examine a small subset of the discharge reports from each provider over an extended period of time. The results from the samples can be useful in drawing conclusions about the quality outcomes of care for each provider.

102. A: In this scenario, the first question would be answered with a simple yes or no option, which is considered nominal because they are categorical data with no natural order. However, a numbering system may be used for calculation purposes (e.g., no = 0, yes = 1). The total number of hours spent sleeping on the same day that alcohol was consumed is considered ordinal. These options have a natural order (e.g., 0–3 = little sleep, 4–6 = a moderate amount of sleep, 7–9 = a full night's rest). The temperature of an individual is considered interval data because it is continuous data that does not have a true zero value.

103. C: Extract, transform, and load is the most widely used data integration technique for big data systems. This integration technique pulls data from its source systems, copies them and then converts them by duplication or combining them into other data. After data are extracted and transformed, they can be loaded into the target database.

104. B: A data dictionary controls whether or not an input mask should be used and tells a database the format that should be used to display the number. For example, a mask for phone numbers may appear in the system or may be entered as (123) 456-7890. Masks are commonly used to format social security numbers (XXX-XX-XXXX) and dates (MM/DD/YY).

105. A: When revisions have to be made to clinical documentation, healthcare professionals must use caution ensuring to make edits in the original record using amendments. Original information should never be deleted or rewritten. After changes have been made, the individual who made the modifications must digitally sign the entry and include the person's credentials and the date and time that the changes were made.

106. D: Patients have the right to request amendments to PHI included in the designated record set. Reasonable requests made regarding erroneous medical record documentation can be resolved. However, the patient may be required to make their request in writing and support the reason for the amendment. Requests made could be denied if the PHI is not part of the designated record set, was not created by the covered entity, if the record is not available for inspection, or if the documentation is complete and accurate.

107. A: According to the HIPAA Privacy Rule, compound authorizations can only be combined with another type of permission for the same research study. For example, an authorization form that combines the use or disclosure of PHI and consents to receive treatment. In this scenario, a patient plans on participating in a different clinical trial. Therefore, the principal investigator should obtain an updated authorization form from the patient before moving forward.

108. B: Frequently referred to as "data about data," metadata are used to increase the effectiveness of data. Metadata describes the "who, what, where, when, how, and why" of data, making it easier to locate and work with that data. Metadata enhance data value and reuse by providing important context for data management.

109. A: Duplicate MPI entries are the most common data quality issue, occurring when a patient has more than one unique identifier (i.e., medical record number). Duplicate medical records can negatively impact data accuracy, create patient safety risks, and result in financial loss. Therefore, registration staff must validate a patient's identity and ensure that the patient is not already registered in the MPI under a nickname, as shown in this question.

110. D: Data governance encompasses oversight functions and decision-making authority over data-related matters. Data governance outlines, implements, and enforces policies, procedures, structures, and standards that define how data are captured, stored, and retrieved. A data governance plan helps organizations coordinate and align the management of information to support strategic business goals.

111. D: This scenario describes a context-based access control (CBAC) security mechanism. This security mechanism is the most stringent because it is an application-specific constraint that factors user context in addition to the attributes of the resource being accessed. Consider the following scenario: An intensive care unit requires ID badge access to enter, and the computers in this secured area likely house applications specific to this level of care. The CBAC system checks to ensure that the access originated from the precise location where the intensive care unit is located in the facility and makes sure that the login information is authenticated before allowing access to the user.

112. B: The HITECH Act implemented changes to the accounting of disclosures. Under this rule, individuals have the right to receive an accounting of disclosures made during the past 3 years as opposed to the 6 years required under the HIPAA Privacy Rule.

113. B: When it comes to effectively managing risks, organizations have the option to avoid, mitigate, transfer, and accept the risk. When the findings of a risk analysis uncover risks, avoidance is no longer a viable option because it has already occurred. In this situation, the organization should consider carrying out the following methods:

- Mitigate—Reduce or Eliminate the risk by implementing controls.
- Transfer—Outsource or Insure the risk against any potential losses.
- Accept—Understand and acknowledge that residual risks will exist and take no action to resolve, transfer, or mitigate risks.

It is recommended that all risks be evaluated and that no risks are left unaddressed.

114. B: The Data Use and Reciprocal Support Agreement is a legally binding contract that defines the requirements for participation in the eHealth Exchange national network. This agreement draws from federal and local laws detailing the obligations/responsibilities and sanctions for contract violations, which apply to all participating members.

115. C: A *qui tam relator* can be anyone (patients, competitors, or employees) who submits a claim to the federal government based on their knowledge or evidence of fraudulent activities. These individuals, also known as whistleblowers, are protected under the Federal False Claims Act and are safe from harassment, demotion, termination, or discrimination from their company after filing a lawsuit. *Qui tam relators* receive a minimum of 15% of any money recovered by the government related to fraudulent activities.

116. C: To improve data integrity, the change needed to be applied to the data descriptors would be requiring acceptable data field values. The definition of admission date is clear and concise. Using *date* as the data type is appropriate; the length of 15 characters is also acceptable if the date is written in full (i.e., September 24, 2014). It is also necessary to require this field so that this crucial information is not forgotten or missed during the data collection process. Not requiring acceptable data values could result in the entry of dates that have already passed, are in the future, or are nonexistent.

117. C: A virtual private network (VPN) uses tunneling to establish a secure connection so remote users can safely access their organization's private network. VPNs encrypt data being sent and decrypt data being received in order to avoid interception by unauthorized users. VPNs hide IP addresses and enhance online privacy while providing anonymity.

118. D: This table has a formatting error of missing column headings. For productivity reports to be effective, they must be developed clearly and concisely. The numbers in each column lack context, making it difficult to understand what is being measured or to determine what these values represent. Adding column headings will allow readers to properly interpret the data.

119. C: The nurse would have been able to access her son's medical record after he received his appendectomy because at that time he was a minor. However, Anne's son has reached the age of majority and is now considered an adult. Therefore, Anne no longer has the right to access her son's medical records without permission from him in the form of a signed authorization ROI form designating that she can obtain a copy of his medical record.

120. A: A disease index can be used to identify any reportable case of cancer over a particular period. The disease index consists of a list of diagnosis codes for patients discharged from a healthcare facility, created from compiled results of abstracting ICD-10-CM diagnosis codes. Patients who match this criterion can easily be identified.

121. B: Interoperability is a term used to describe the ability of different IT systems to accurately and securely exchange information without experiencing glitches or loss of data integrity. Interoperability of various health IT applications can improve patient outcomes, can streamline and optimize operations, and could reduce costs by eliminating redundant testing.

122. D: A business associate agreement (BAA) is a contract between a covered entity and a business associate that establishes permitted uses and disclosures of PHI. BAAs often define permissible and impermissible uses and disclosures, and they outline liability consequences when the agreement is breached. Once these agreements are created, they should be developed into clearly defined operational policies.

123. C: Of the options listed, all of these situations would be permitted by HIPAA's Privacy Rule except releasing the names and phone numbers of diabetic patients to a pharmaceutical company without acquiring authorization from the patient(s) or their representative(s) first. A healthcare provider must obtain authorized consent from the individual before disclosing any PHI to any outside entities who plan to use the information for marketing purposes.

124. D: Healthcare organizations must comply with the Conditions of Participation to participate in and receive payments from the Medicare and Medicaid programs. Deemed status can be achieved by meeting/exceeding Medicare and Medicaid requirements or displaying compliance during CMS, accrediting body, or state agency surveys.

125. B: When a user accesses the ePHI of patients with the same last name, a trigger flag is activated, alerting the internal audit team of suspicious electronic activity. Intentionally and inappropriately accessing information that is not for a work-related purpose constitutes a breach of confidentiality. However, each instance may require closer inspection because an employee with a common last name could be accessing the medical records of a patient with the same last name yet have no relation to them.

126. B: Outsourcing has become a popular alternate staffing option that organizations have taken advantage of in recent years. Workers are hired from third parties within the country or overseas to accomplish work tasks remotely and help an organization achieve its business goals. Outsourcing is often seen as a cost-effective way to improve business efficiency, and it allows organizations to work with more expansive talent pool ranges.

127. D: A champion is an individual who is dedicated to improving and facilitating change within their organization. Champions often focus on gaps in performance, improving standards, and promoting new ideas. This is a crucial job position that improves morale through the encouragement and motivation of others to ensure that the organization is operating optimally.

128. A: The recommended action would be to ensure that any records involved in pending litigation or belonging to minors are examined more closely. Organizations must adhere to the retention guidelines that allow for the longest period of time whether that be federal or state statues or accreditation standards. Each state's retention periods vary, so it is essential to determine the most stringent retention requirements in your area before destroying any medical records. Records being stored that are involved in pending litigation should be retained until the legal proceedings come to an end. Also, the records of minors must be retained until the minor reaches the age of majority, which can also vary considerably from state to state.

129. B: Telehealth and telemedicine services integrate videoconferencing with other technologies to support convenient interactive meetings between patients and providers. Telehealth can provide long-distance medical care to underserved populations in a timely fashion. Smart wearable devices can monitor vital signs and blood sugar levels, allowing providers to track patients' progress over time and help manage their conditions.

130. D: P-values are calculated from statistical tests and are used in hypothesis testing to decide whether to reject the null hypothesis. If a p-value is equivalent to or less than the selected significance level, reject the null hypothesis.

131. C: Accountable care organizations, patient-centered medical homes, and bundled payments (episode based) are models under the value-based purchasing program.

- Accountable care organizations comprise a group of physicians or hospitals that provide Medicare beneficiaries with high-quality coordinated care.
- Patient-centered medical homes deliver comprehensive/coordinated care in a centralized setting to manage the various needs of patients. They focus on improving patient outcomes, safety, staff experiences, and system efficiency.
- Bundled payments collectively reimburse providers based on the expected costs associated with treating certain conditions that could span various settings of care and include different providers or require multiple procedures.

132. B: Delinquent records refer to medical records that are not completed in a specified time frame. Attending physicians have a responsibility to ensure the timely completion of medical records. Delinquent records present patient safety, legal, compliance, and financial risks. A missing physician signature is a common issue that leaves medical records incomplete.

133. B: A network of data stewards has the responsibility and accountability of ensuring data quality and that the agreed-upon metrics are maintained on a continual basis. These individuals are usually appointed for data within their specific domain; their duties can include, but are not limited to, developing data definitions, adhering to privacy standards, monitoring data quality, and testing security procedures.

134. D: Billing all patients for the highest level of evaluation and management despite actually providing this level of care to every patient would be considered upcoding. This is fraudulent activity. The level of evaluation and management codes should be based on the patient's actual medical condition and should reflect the time and detailed extent of the encounter.

135. A: When unsecured PHI is accessed or released without the patient's consent, this is considered a breach of privacy and security. Breach notification reporting requirements mandate that when 500 or more individuals have been affected, the covered entity and its business associates must immediately report the breach to the impacted individuals, the secretary of HHS, and the local media.

136. A: Normalization consists of organizing data in databases by creating tables and establishing relationships between the tables designed to make the database more flexible. Normalization helps reduce redundancies or inconsistent dependencies and ultimately improves data quality. An example of normalization is entering a patient's first and last names into separate fields.

137. B: When a confirmed case of mpox is identified by a healthcare provider, it must be reported immediately or at least within 24 hours by calling the applicable local health department. Elements that should be reported include, but are not limited to, the individual's name, address, phone number, gender, test result, the attending physician's name, and the Clinical Laboratory Improvement Amendments (CLIA) number (which shows that the laboratory meets CMS quality standards) of the clinical laboratory facility that performed the testing.

138. B: Assessing productivity levels across various employee coders who work on cases from different departments or have varying employment statuses can be challenging. At first glance, Kaleigh looks to be completing the most coding cases per day; however, emergency department cases often require the least amount of time to code. Inpatient coding is the most complex, taking substantially more time to complete because coders must review longer reports that cover a full range of services. Therefore, Daniel and Hobart would be expected to complete significantly fewer charts compared to the other coders. This example shows that it can sometimes be difficult to make conclusions based on productivity standard reports without having the necessary background information.

139. D: The quality committee should not ignore its finding that almost half of the organization's databases do not have an associated data dictionary. Establishing a policy and the associated standards on the need for and use of data dictionaries is an essential first step for the committee to take. After the standards and policy are put in place, employee training and memorandums can be created and delivered to inform and educate workforce members on the importance and value of data dictionaries whether they are database specific or organization-wide.

140. D: A record locator service helps point out where patient records might be located by using criteria such as the geographic area, personal ID, data type, or other information. A record locator service query indicates where a patient's data are likely to be stored and allows providers to strategically retrieve records that match the demographic information in the query.

141. B: The Joint Commission requires a history and physical examination to be incorporated into a patient's medical record before any surgery or procedure that involves the administration of anesthesia is conducted. The only exception to this standard is emergency situations in which delays in care could be detrimental to the patient's condition.

142. C: The Uniform Data System (UDS) is an annual reporting system consisting of various recommended data elements such as staffing, care utilization, patient demographics, disparities in health outcomes, indicators of quality care, and revenue. These data elements use consistent definitions to provide standardized information about the operations and performance of healthcare centers that render services to vulnerable populations or underserved communities. The UDS ensures compliance with regulatory requirements, identifies trends over time, and keeps track of program effectiveness.

143. C: The Hospital-Issued Notice of Noncoverage (HINN) form can be provided to Medicare beneficiaries before or at admission and any point during their hospital stay. Of the options listed, the lack of preauthorization is not a valid reason to provide a patient with a HINN.

144. B: All variances related to accounting are referred to as either favorable or unfavorable. In this scenario, the cost of the HIM department's printer was less than the budgeted amount, meaning that the department incurred a lower price than expected (a favorable variance). Any budget variances, whether favorable or unfavorable, should always be identified and explained to the HIM director or chief financial officer.

145. B: Data mining, also known as knowledge discovery in database, uses sophisticated technology to sort through an organization's structured data to uncover unusual or hidden patterns. Data mining is based on mathematical methods and can contribute to making optimal business decisions, detecting fraud, or forecasting future trends.

146. C: All employees, regardless of their position within a healthcare facility, should receive HIPAA compliance training within a reasonable period after joining the workforce. This usually occurs during their initial orientation period and continues periodically throughout their employment. This training usually reinforces knowledge on topics such as the Privacy or Security Rules, breach notifications, patient rights, preventing HIPAA violations, rules for disclosures, and more.

147. B: *Subpoena duces tecum* is a Latin term that means "you shall bring with you." This subpoena compels an individual to bring records to a legal proceeding. Therefore, Abigail will be responsible for delivering the requested documents or appearing in person to present such evidence. Abigail will not be required to provide oral testimony unless a *subpoena ad testificandum* accompanies the *subpoena duces tecum*.

148. D: When multiple lacerations in the same anatomic location are repaired, the length of each laceration should be summed, and a single CPT code should be reported. However, if the lacerations were located in different anatomic locations of the body, then multiple CPT codes can be used to report each laceration.

149. A: For doctors to provide treatment or services to patients, they must first be deemed reasonable and necessary for the related diagnosis. In this case, the clinical documentation lacks medical necessity. Medical records must support the services provided. Therefore, the chest x-ray would not be covered by the patient's insurance company because this procedure is not related to the leg pain that the individual was experiencing.

150. C: Data consistency is the dimension of data quality absent from Mr. Brown's medical record. In this scenario, the inconsistencies of the patient's date of birth may cause Mr. Brown's medical record to be erroneously filed under another patient's chart—or a separate record (under a different medical record number) could be created for Mr. Brown due to the incorrect date of birth. If data quality is not consistent throughout a medical record, it can present dangers such as inaccuracies, medical errors, duplicate testing, or other adverse events.

151. A: Automated reviews performed by recovery audit contractors can detect errors and deny payments without having to review the medical documentation. In this case, duplicate billing for two appendectomies on the same day for the same patient could be easily identified as a potential improper payment.

152. A: Addressing gaps in care will likely improve health outcomes. Leveraging technology can help track data trends, optimize workflows, and foster better coordinated care. Identifying high-risk patients allows providers to implement preventative care measures to reduce the impacts of diseases or chronic medical conditions. These options would all contribute to increasing the overall quality of care. Because giving value-based care rewards healthcare organizations for the quality of services provided to patients, charging based on the quantity of services rendered would not be considered a successful strategy.

153. A: Super users are typically staff members who will eventually be end users and receive additional training on systems so they can help train other employees and stay updated. Appointing super users is beneficial for users and organizations: It can promote employee growth and equip the facility with frontline workers from whom other end users can seek guidance when necessary.

154. A: The HIPAA Privacy Rule requires covered entities to provide individuals with access to their PHI upon request. This rule also specifies that individuals have the right to access their PHI for as long as the information is maintained by the entity or by a business associate.

155. D: This is an example of a leading query because the coder suggests a new diagnosis not specified in the medical record documentation. Using open-ended query methods that include multiple-choice options is more likely to result in an accurate code selection instead of suggesting a new diagnosis or procedure that is not supported in the clinical documentation. Also, leading queries must not be performed with the intention of improving reimbursement amounts.

156. D: Healthcare providers have a responsibility to report cases of diseases that are considered to be important to public health so that outbreaks can be tracked and controlled. The National Notifiable Diseases Surveillance System mandates that healthcare providers report notifiable diseases at the local, state, and national levels. The list of notifiable diseases can vary over time and from state to state—but, of the options listed, diabetes mellitus would not be considered a reportable disease.

157. C: Unbundling is a form of medical billing fraud by using multiple procedure codes that could have been coded as a single bundled procedure. Unbundling is an illegal practice that is often done with the intention of increasing reimbursement. In this scenario, one code (37760) should have been used to represent the bundled services included in the code instead of reporting the separate codes 37760 and 15271. The skin graft described in code 15271 is already included in code 37760.

158. C: Automatic logoff capabilities of computers are considered a technical safeguard used to protect and control access to PHI. Physical safeguards are concerned with protecting the environment, information systems, and equipment from environmental hazards and unauthorized intrusion.

159. C: Based on the pie chart, Medicare patients make up half (200) of the individuals who have received the flu vaccine is the most accurate statement. We cannot determine if uninsured patients are choosing not to receive the shot or if the flu vaccine is mandated by Medicare and Medicaid. Also, based on these findings, it is reasonable to surmise that a patient's insurance status could have some impact on their ability to receive the flu vaccine.

160. D: A histogram is used to summarize and display frequency distributions of continuous data. Numeric values are broken down into bins spanning each bar, while the height of each bar represents the density of each binned group. Histograms are especially useful when dealing with large data sets, and they can help detect any gaps or outliers within the data.

161. D: AHIMA recommends that after records reach their retention period end date, they must be destroyed so that the information contained therein cannot be reconstructed. A certificate of destruction (COD) is a document created to confirm that sensitive materials have been destroyed properly. Typical elements of a COD include, but are not limited to, the date of destruction, a description of the disposed-of records, the method of destruction used, and a statement saying that the records were destroyed in the normal course of business. The COD should be kept permanently to serve as evidence that records were destroyed in compliance with regulations, which protects the entity in the event of legal action.

162. B: Recruitment is the act of soliciting and assessing potential candidates to fill staff openings. An organization's human resources department often conducts the recruitment process. However, those in supervisory or managerial roles can also perform this activity. The goal of recruitment is to find individuals best suited to fill vacant positions and ensure that they are qualified for those roles.

163. C: Employee orientation occurs immediately after a person is hired and is used to welcome/introduce individuals to their new workplace. A review of organizational culture, policies, practices, and procedures can be expected during this process. Depending on the organization and job role, orientation can last from a single day to a week and can include facility tours and information regarding benefits, training, and mentoring.

164. A: The Uniform Hospital Discharge Data Set (UHDDS) is an inpatient data set incorporated into federal law used to report and compare performance, reimbursement rates, or other aspects of delivered healthcare services. This core data set for inpatient admissions is collected for the Medicare and Medicaid programs from discharge reports. Major patient-specific elements of the UHDDS include, but are not limited to, the principal diagnosis; procedures performed; and the age, sex, and race of a patient. In addition to hospitals, nursing homes, rehabilitation centers, psychiatric facilities, home health providers, and payers have also begun using the UHDDS.

165. D: Covered entities and the business associates who they contract with have a responsibility to properly train all of their workforce members regarding PHI policies and procedures. HIPAA training is an administrative requirement of the Privacy Rule and an administrative safeguard of the Security Rule. It is mandatory to continuously train all individuals, whether or not they have access to PHI.

166. A: Firewall systems include hardware and software devices designed to protect networks from unauthorized intrusion. Commonly, these devices are located between a healthcare entity's internal network and the internet. Although firewalls reduce the likelihood of unauthorized access, they are not considered effective in preventing all possible types of attacks on healthcare systems.

167. D: The Breach Notification Rule requires covered entities and business associates to have policies, procedures, and processes in place to inspect the uses and disclosures of PHI to determine if a breach has occurred. Any time that an individual's PHI has been breached, a covered entity must notify the affected individual with a written notice no later than 60 days after the discovery of the breach.

168. D: Simulations are a training approach used to replicate real-world scenarios that allow individuals to practice various skills in a carefully controlled setting (virtually or in person). Trainees' actions can be monitored to ensure that they can perform clinical procedures without putting patients at risk if errors are committed. Simulations are a highly effective way for new healthcare professionals to enhance their overall clinical knowledge, they allow educators to track competency, and they assist medical students in safely transitioning into healthcare environments.

169. B: Patient falls, adverse medication reactions, wrong surgery site errors, and hospital-acquired conditions are all considered sentinel events that could result in harm to patients or even death. According to the table, each measure has decreased in frequency, which is considered a positive direction in performance. Decreasing the percentage of these adverse events would mean that the quality of care has improved between the third and fourth quarters.

170. B: Based on the options listed, the correct codes are I10 and I51.5. Code I10 indicates essential (primary) hypertension (high blood pressure), and code I51.5 indicates myocardial degeneration of the heart.

171. B: Clinical documentation improvement (CDI) consists of carefully reviewing medical records to determine if any missing, conflicting, or nonspecific information can be detected. The goal of CDI is to achieve an accurate assignment of diagnosis and procedure code(s) and ensure that the clinical documentation supports the selected codes, reflects the level of services rendered to patients, and captures the clinical complexity of the reported condition(s). CDI has many benefits, including, but not limited to, improving patient care, health outcomes, and reimbursement rates and meeting compliance standards.

172. A: Forming, storming, norming, and performing (FSNP) are the stages of development as teams progress.

- Forming is the initial creation of the team. During this stage, members set clear goals/expectations and orient themselves to the project task(s).
- Storming is the second stage and is considered the most difficult. Frustrations often stem from conflicts, confusion, and concerns about meeting goals, which can cause tension.
- Norming is the stage during project development in which team members learn to work together and appreciate each other's strengths. Discrepancies are resolved through constructive criticism, and productivity is increased through a shift in harmonious working relationships.
- Performing is the final stage, in which problem solving is used to achieve shared goals. The team is operating at its full potential, and achievements/goals are celebrated.

173. B: Aggregate data refer to the collection of data on large populations of individuals from multiple sources without revealing any individually identifiable information on said individuals. In this scenario, information was extracted from patients' medical records and combined to develop cohesive information regarding groups of patients. Aggregate data can be used to summarize data sets, answer analytical questions, and assist with business processes.

174. B: To help individuals make informed decisions, providers are instructed to issue an advanced Beneficiary Notice of Noncoverage (ABN) form to inform patients of their financial responsibility when services are believed to not be covered by Medicare due to local or national coverage determinations. ABNs can be issued due to experimental services, a service that is not indicated for the diagnosis, or if the service exceeds the amount allowed during a specific period for that diagnosis.

175. D: This security breach could have been prevented if the hospital handled the electronic media properly by implementing device and media controls. Four implementation specifications are included in HIPAA's device and media controls, including disposal, media reuse, accountability, and data backup and storage. This instance refers to media reuse; the hospital should have closely monitored the removal of hardware containing ePHI from their facility because, otherwise, it could present serious privacy and security risks.

176. A: Ranging from 0 to 100, the TPS encompasses summed weighted domain scores from clinical outcomes, person/community engagement, safety, efficiency, and cost reduction. A higher TPS is better than a lower one because every point increase in the TPS will result in increased payments by a portion of holdback dollars.

177. C: Information blocking occurs when healthcare providers, health IT developers, or HIEs limit, restrict, or interfere with the access, exchange, and use of electronic health information. According to the 2020 Cures Act Final Rule, the eight exceptions to not fulfilling a request include security, privacy, health IT performance, preventing harm, infeasibility, licensing, fees, and content/manner. In this case, the provider knows that disabling his staff from having the ability to share any electronic health information is unreasonable and would be considered information blocking.

178. C: Often formulated by high-level management personnel, strategic plans are used to assess a changing healthcare environment and create a vision for its future state. These plans incorporate a company's mission/vision statements and set specific goals. This long-term direction often spans a 3–5-year period.

179. A: A pie chart is the most efficient data display tool to compare values or proportions of subgroups to an entire data set. The data in pie charts are usually displayed as percentages or decimals, and the total of all the subgroups should always equal 100 percent.

180. B: After data have been posted to a patient's account, internal auditing systems called scrubbers are used to review the generated claim for completeness and accuracy. Claim scrubbers identify and eliminate coding errors that help reduce the number of denied claims by auditing them before they are sent to insurance companies.

181. D: A master patient index (MPI) is used to identify patients across separate clinical, administrative, and financial systems by linking them to a single identifier (usually a medical record number). Some of the recommended core elements for the MPI include, but are not limited to, the patient's first and last name, address, date of birth, social security number, medical record number, gender, and admission/discharge dates.

182. D: The hybrid architectural model is a mixture of centralized and decentralized (federated) HIE models. Participants can query centralized databases and warehouses tethered to the HIE. The decentralized aspect provides increased security and data redundancy because it remains connected to the individual participants. The hybrid model incorporates the best aspects of these two models.

183. C: The unique patient identifier, also known as a patient ID or medical record number, is considered the most reliable. This number is assigned during the registration process. The other options are not optimal because patients can share an address, date of birth, and last name with other patients. A patient ID cannot be shared and is unique to individual patients.

184. B: Information governance policies and procedures are essential to guiding data management processes within an organization. Policies and procedures should include, but are not limited to, components such as the organization's name, date of creation, title, policy statement, scope, responsible parties, definitions, and references. Policies and procedures should avoid using legalese that may be difficult to understand.

185. D: Practice management systems can integrate and manage scheduling, administrative, billing, and registration functions across an organization. Practice management software can be used in medical practices of any size. They have many benefits including reducing errors, saving staff time, processing reimbursement more quickly, and allowing easier access to EHRs.

186. A: Admit, discharge, and transfer (ADT) systems track patients from their arrival at a healthcare organization until discharge. Information is stored on these systems and can be shared with other facilities, including the patient's name, age, medical record number, and contact information. ADT notifications can be shared with different care team members, which can ultimately improve the quality of patient care/coordination, increase hospital productivity, and enhance the use of patient histories.

187. A: Data governance should not be considered a one-time project. Instead, data governance should be an iterative process that is done continuously. Other data governance functions include, but are not limited to, enforcing data security policies, increasing end users' data literacy and skills, managing enterprise data, and influencing the behaviors of stakeholders toward efficient use of data to meet organizational goals.

188. A: HIPAA is a federal law that requires medical records to be maintained for 6 years. However, the laws for retention can vary by state and may be lengthier. The HIM professional should defer to the longest retention period requirements.

189. C: Various algorithms are used to determine the probability of duplicate medical records existing throughout an EMPI that reference patients in two or more integrated healthcare facilities.

- Rules-based algorithms assign weights to particular data elements and make comparisons of records based on the aggregated score.
- Probabilistic algorithms are considered the most effective. These algorithms use complex mathematical formulas to analyze MPI data to determine the probability of data matches based on matched weight probabilities of the attribute values of data elements.
- Deterministic algorithms require an exact or near match of combined data elements such as name, DOB, SSN, etc.

How to Overcome Test Anxiety

Just the thought of taking a test is enough to make most people a little nervous. A test is an important event that can have a long-term impact on your future, so it's important to take it seriously and it's natural to feel anxious about performing well. But just because anxiety is normal, that doesn't mean that it's helpful in test taking, or that you should simply accept it as part of your life. Anxiety can have a variety of effects. These effects can be mild, like making you feel slightly nervous, or severe, like blocking your ability to focus or remember even a simple detail.

If you experience test anxiety—whether severe or mild—it's important to know how to beat it. To discover this, first you need to understand what causes test anxiety.

Causes of Test Anxiety

While we often think of anxiety as an uncontrollable emotional state, it can actually be caused by simple, practical things. One of the most common causes of test anxiety is that a person does not feel adequately prepared for their test. This feeling can be the result of many different issues such as poor study habits or lack of organization, but the most common culprit is time management. Starting to study too late, failing to organize your study time to cover all of the material, or being distracted while you study will mean that you're not well prepared for the test. This may lead to cramming the night before, which will cause you to be physically and mentally exhausted for the test. Poor time management also contributes to feelings of stress, fear, and hopelessness as you realize you are not well prepared but don't know what to do about it.

Other times, test anxiety is not related to your preparation for the test but comes from unresolved fear. This may be a past failure on a test, or poor performance on tests in general. It may come from comparing yourself to others who seem to be performing better or from the stress of living up to expectations. Anxiety may be driven by fears of the future—how failure on this test would affect your educational and career goals. These fears are often completely irrational, but they can still negatively impact your test performance.

> **Review Video: 3 Reasons You Have Test Anxiety**
> Visit mometrix.com/academy and enter code: 428468

Elements of Test Anxiety

As mentioned earlier, test anxiety is considered to be an emotional state, but it has physical and mental components as well. Sometimes you may not even realize that you are suffering from test anxiety until you notice the physical symptoms. These can include trembling hands, rapid heartbeat, sweating, nausea, and tense muscles. Extreme anxiety may lead to fainting or vomiting. Obviously, any of these symptoms can have a negative impact on testing. It is important to recognize them as soon as they begin to occur so that you can address the problem before it damages your performance.

> **Review Video: 3 Ways to Tell You Have Test Anxiety**
> Visit mometrix.com/academy and enter code: 927847

The mental components of test anxiety include trouble focusing and inability to remember learned information. During a test, your mind is on high alert, which can help you recall information and stay focused for an extended period of time. However, anxiety interferes with your mind's natural processes, causing you to blank out, even on the questions you know well. The strain of testing during anxiety makes it difficult to stay focused, especially on a test that may take several hours. Extreme anxiety can take a huge mental toll, making it difficult not only to recall test information but even to understand the test questions or pull your thoughts together.

> **Review Video: How Test Anxiety Affects Memory**
> Visit mometrix.com/academy and enter code: 609003

Effects of Test Anxiety

Test anxiety is like a disease—if left untreated, it will get progressively worse. Anxiety leads to poor performance, and this reinforces the feelings of fear and failure, which in turn lead to poor performances on subsequent tests. It can grow from a mild nervousness to a crippling condition. If allowed to progress, test anxiety can have a big impact on your schooling, and consequently on your future.

Test anxiety can spread to other parts of your life. Anxiety on tests can become anxiety in any stressful situation, and blanking on a test can turn into panicking in a job situation. But fortunately, you don't have to let anxiety rule your testing and determine your grades. There are a number of relatively simple steps you can take to move past anxiety and function normally on a test and in the rest of life.

> **Review Video: How Test Anxiety Impacts Your Grades**
> Visit mometrix.com/academy and enter code: 939819

Physical Steps for Beating Test Anxiety

While test anxiety is a serious problem, the good news is that it can be overcome. It doesn't have to control your ability to think and remember information. While it may take time, you can begin taking steps today to beat anxiety.

Just as your first hint that you may be struggling with anxiety comes from the physical symptoms, the first step to treating it is also physical. Rest is crucial for having a clear, strong mind. If you are tired, it is much easier to give in to anxiety. But if you establish good sleep habits, your body and mind will be ready to perform optimally, without the strain of exhaustion. Additionally, sleeping well helps you to retain information better, so you're more likely to recall the answers when you see the test questions.

Getting good sleep means more than going to bed on time. It's important to allow your brain time to relax. Take study breaks from time to time so it doesn't get overworked, and don't study right before bed. Take time to rest your mind before trying to rest your body, or you may find it difficult to fall asleep.

> **Review Video: The Importance of Sleep for Your Brain**
> Visit mometrix.com/academy and enter code: 319338

Along with sleep, other aspects of physical health are important in preparing for a test. Good nutrition is vital for good brain function. Sugary foods and drinks may give a burst of energy but this burst is followed by a crash, both physically and emotionally. Instead, fuel your body with protein and vitamin-rich foods.

Also, drink plenty of water. Dehydration can lead to headaches and exhaustion, especially if your brain is already under stress from the rigors of the test. Particularly if your test is a long one, drink water during the breaks. And if possible, take an energy-boosting snack to eat between sections.

> **Review Video: How Diet Can Affect your Mood**
> Visit mometrix.com/academy and enter code: 624317

Along with sleep and diet, a third important part of physical health is exercise. Maintaining a steady workout schedule is helpful, but even taking 5-minute study breaks to walk can help get your blood pumping faster and clear your head. Exercise also releases endorphins, which contribute to a positive feeling and can help combat test anxiety.

When you nurture your physical health, you are also contributing to your mental health. If your body is healthy, your mind is much more likely to be healthy as well. So take time to rest, nourish your body with healthy food and water, and get moving as much as possible. Taking these physical steps will make you stronger and more able to take the mental steps necessary to overcome test anxiety.

Mental Steps for Beating Test Anxiety

Working on the mental side of test anxiety can be more challenging, but as with the physical side, there are clear steps you can take to overcome it. As mentioned earlier, test anxiety often stems from lack of preparation, so the obvious solution is to prepare for the test. Effective studying may be the most important weapon you have for beating test anxiety, but you can and should employ several other mental tools to combat fear.

First, boost your confidence by reminding yourself of past success—tests or projects that you aced. If you're putting as much effort into preparing for this test as you did for those, there's no reason you should expect to fail here. Work hard to prepare; then trust your preparation.

Second, surround yourself with encouraging people. It can be helpful to find a study group, but be sure that the people you're around will encourage a positive attitude. If you spend time with others who are anxious or cynical, this will only contribute to your own anxiety. Look for others who are motivated to study hard from a desire to succeed, not from a fear of failure.

Third, reward yourself. A test is physically and mentally tiring, even without anxiety, and it can be helpful to have something to look forward to. Plan an activity following the test, regardless of the outcome, such as going to a movie or getting ice cream.

When you are taking the test, if you find yourself beginning to feel anxious, remind yourself that you know the material. Visualize successfully completing the test. Then take a few deep, relaxing breaths and return to it. Work through the questions carefully but with confidence, knowing that you are capable of succeeding.

Developing a healthy mental approach to test taking will also aid in other areas of life. Test anxiety affects more than just the actual test—it can be damaging to your mental health and even contribute to depression. It's important to beat test anxiety before it becomes a problem for more than testing.

> **Review Video: Test Anxiety and Depression**
> Visit mometrix.com/academy and enter code: 904704

Study Strategy

Being prepared for the test is necessary to combat anxiety, but what does being prepared look like? You may study for hours on end and still not feel prepared. What you need is a strategy for test prep. The next few pages outline our recommended steps to help you plan out and conquer the challenge of preparation.

STEP 1: SCOPE OUT THE TEST

Learn everything you can about the format (multiple choice, essay, etc.) and what will be on the test. Gather any study materials, course outlines, or sample exams that may be available. Not only will this help you to prepare, but knowing what to expect can help to alleviate test anxiety.

STEP 2: MAP OUT THE MATERIAL

Look through the textbook or study guide and make note of how many chapters or sections it has. Then divide these over the time you have. For example, if a book has 15 chapters and you have five days to study, you need to cover three chapters each day. Even better, if you have the time, leave an extra day at the end for overall review after you have gone through the material in depth.

If time is limited, you may need to prioritize the material. Look through it and make note of which sections you think you already have a good grasp on, and which need review. While you are studying, skim quickly through the familiar sections and take more time on the challenging parts. Write out your plan so you don't get lost as you go. Having a written plan also helps you feel more in control of the study, so anxiety is less likely to arise from feeling overwhelmed at the amount to cover.

STEP 3: GATHER YOUR TOOLS

Decide what study method works best for you. Do you prefer to highlight in the book as you study and then go back over the highlighted portions? Or do you type out notes of the important information? Or is it helpful to make flashcards that you can carry with you? Assemble the pens, index cards, highlighters, post-it notes, and any other materials you may need so you won't be distracted by getting up to find things while you study.

If you're having a hard time retaining the information or organizing your notes, experiment with different methods. For example, try color-coding by subject with colored pens, highlighters, or post-it notes. If you learn better by hearing, try recording yourself reading your notes so you can listen while in the car, working out, or simply sitting at your desk. Ask a friend to quiz you from your flashcards, or try teaching someone the material to solidify it in your mind.

STEP 4: CREATE YOUR ENVIRONMENT

It's important to avoid distractions while you study. This includes both the obvious distractions like visitors and the subtle distractions like an uncomfortable chair (or a too-comfortable couch that makes you want to fall asleep). Set up the best study environment possible: good lighting and a comfortable work area. If background music helps you focus, you may want to turn it on, but otherwise keep the room quiet. If you are using a computer to take notes, be sure you don't have any other windows open, especially applications like social media, games, or anything else that could distract you. Silence your phone and turn off notifications. Be sure to keep water close by so you stay hydrated while you study (but avoid unhealthy drinks and snacks).

Also, take into account the best time of day to study. Are you freshest first thing in the morning? Try to set aside some time then to work through the material. Is your mind clearer in the afternoon or evening? Schedule your study session then. Another method is to study at the same time of day that you will take the test, so that your brain gets used to working on the material at that time and will be ready to focus at test time.

Step 5: Study!

Once you have done all the study preparation, it's time to settle into the actual studying. Sit down, take a few moments to settle your mind so you can focus, and begin to follow your study plan. Don't give in to distractions or let yourself procrastinate. This is your time to prepare so you'll be ready to fearlessly approach the test. Make the most of the time and stay focused.

Of course, you don't want to burn out. If you study too long you may find that you're not retaining the information very well. Take regular study breaks. For example, taking five minutes out of every hour to walk briskly, breathing deeply and swinging your arms, can help your mind stay fresh.

As you get to the end of each chapter or section, it's a good idea to do a quick review. Remind yourself of what you learned and work on any difficult parts. When you feel that you've mastered the material, move on to the next part. At the end of your study session, briefly skim through your notes again.

But while review is helpful, cramming last minute is NOT. If at all possible, work ahead so that you won't need to fit all your study into the last day. Cramming overloads your brain with more information than it can process and retain, and your tired mind may struggle to recall even previously learned information when it is overwhelmed with last-minute study. Also, the urgent nature of cramming and the stress placed on your brain contribute to anxiety. You'll be more likely to go to the test feeling unprepared and having trouble thinking clearly.

So don't cram, and don't stay up late before the test, even just to review your notes at a leisurely pace. Your brain needs rest more than it needs to go over the information again. In fact, plan to finish your studies by noon or early afternoon the day before the test. Give your brain the rest of the day to relax or focus on other things, and get a good night's sleep. Then you will be fresh for the test and better able to recall what you've studied.

Step 6: Take a practice test

Many courses offer sample tests, either online or in the study materials. This is an excellent resource to check whether you have mastered the material, as well as to prepare for the test format and environment.

Check the test format ahead of time: the number of questions, the type (multiple choice, free response, etc.), and the time limit. Then create a plan for working through them. For example, if you have 30 minutes to take a 60-question test, your limit is 30 seconds per question. Spend less time on the questions you know well so that you can take more time on the difficult ones.

If you have time to take several practice tests, take the first one open book, with no time limit. Work through the questions at your own pace and make sure you fully understand them. Gradually work up to taking a test under test conditions: sit at a desk with all study materials put away and set a timer. Pace yourself to make sure you finish the test with time to spare and go back to check your answers if you have time.

After each test, check your answers. On the questions you missed, be sure you understand why you missed them. Did you misread the question (tests can use tricky wording)? Did you forget the information? Or was it something you hadn't learned? Go back and study any shaky areas that the practice tests reveal.

Taking these tests not only helps with your grade, but also aids in combating test anxiety. If you're already used to the test conditions, you're less likely to worry about it, and working through tests until you're scoring well gives you a confidence boost. Go through the practice tests until you feel comfortable, and then you can go into the test knowing that you're ready for it.

Test Tips

On test day, you should be confident, knowing that you've prepared well and are ready to answer the questions. But aside from preparation, there are several test day strategies you can employ to maximize your performance.

First, as stated before, get a good night's sleep the night before the test (and for several nights before that, if possible). Go into the test with a fresh, alert mind rather than staying up late to study.

Try not to change too much about your normal routine on the day of the test. It's important to eat a nutritious breakfast, but if you normally don't eat breakfast at all, consider eating just a protein bar. If you're a coffee drinker, go ahead and have your normal coffee. Just make sure you time it so that the caffeine doesn't wear off right in the middle of your test. Avoid sugary beverages, and drink enough water to stay hydrated but not so much that you need a restroom break 10 minutes into the test. If your test isn't first thing in the morning, consider going for a walk or doing a light workout before the test to get your blood flowing.

Allow yourself enough time to get ready, and leave for the test with plenty of time to spare so you won't have the anxiety of scrambling to arrive in time. Another reason to be early is to select a good seat. It's helpful to sit away from doors and windows, which can be distracting. Find a good seat, get out your supplies, and settle your mind before the test begins.

When the test begins, start by going over the instructions carefully, even if you already know what to expect. Make sure you avoid any careless mistakes by following the directions.

Then begin working through the questions, pacing yourself as you've practiced. If you're not sure on an answer, don't spend too much time on it, and don't let it shake your confidence. Either skip it and come back later, or eliminate as many wrong answers as possible and guess among the remaining ones. Don't dwell on these questions as you continue—put them out of your mind and focus on what lies ahead.

Be sure to read all of the answer choices, even if you're sure the first one is the right answer. Sometimes you'll find a better one if you keep reading. But don't second-guess yourself if you do immediately know the answer. Your gut instinct is usually right. Don't let test anxiety rob you of the information you know.

If you have time at the end of the test (and if the test format allows), go back and review your answers. Be cautious about changing any, since your first instinct tends to be correct, but make sure you didn't misread any of the questions or accidentally mark the wrong answer choice. Look over any you skipped and make an educated guess.

At the end, leave the test feeling confident. You've done your best, so don't waste time worrying about your performance or wishing you could change anything. Instead, celebrate the successful completion of this test. And finally, use this test to learn how to deal with anxiety even better next time.

> **Review Video: 5 Tips to Beat Test Anxiety**
> Visit mometrix.com/academy and enter code: 570656

Important Qualification

Not all anxiety is created equal. If your test anxiety is causing major issues in your life beyond the classroom or testing center, or if you are experiencing troubling physical symptoms related to your anxiety, it may be a sign of a serious physiological or psychological condition. If this sounds like your situation, we strongly encourage you to seek professional help.

Tell Us Your Story

We at Mometrix would like to extend our heartfelt thanks to you for letting us be a part of your journey. It is an honor to serve people from all walks of life, people like you, who are committed to building the best future they can for themselves.

We know that each person's situation is unique. But we also know that, whether you are a young student or a mother of four, you care about working to make your own life and the lives of those around you better.

That's why we want to hear your story.

We want to know why you're taking this test. We want to know about the trials you've gone through to get here. And we want to know about the successes you've experienced after taking and passing your test.

In addition to your story, which can be an inspiration both to us and to others, we value your feedback. We want to know both what you loved about our book and what you think we can improve on.

The team at Mometrix would be absolutely thrilled to hear from you! So please, send us an email at tellusyourstory@mometrix.com or visit us at mometrix.com/tellusyourstory.php and let's stay in touch.

Additional Bonus Material

Due to our efforts to try to keep this book to a manageable length, we've created a link that will give you access to all of your additional bonus material:

mometrix.com/bonus948/rhia

Made in the USA
Coppell, TX
05 March 2024

29804349R00116